Innovation in Esophageal Surgery

Luigi Bonavina
Editor

Innovation in Esophageal Surgery

Foreword by Tom R. DeMeester

Springer

Editor
Prof. Luigi Bonavina
Department of Biomedical Sciences for Health
Division of General Surgery
University of Milan School of Medicine
IRCCS Policlinico San Donato
San Donato Milanese (Milan)
Italy

ISBN 978-88-470-2468-7 ISBN 978-88-470-2469-4 (eBook)
DOI 10.1007/978-88-470-2469-4
Springer Milan Heidelberg New York Dordrecht London

Library of Congress Control Number: 2012948780

Printed on acid-free paper

Springer is part of Springer Science+Business Media (www.springer.com)

Foreword

The 1983 winter in Omaha, Nebraska was particularly severe. Outside my office window I could see two persons trudging through the deep, newly fallen snow. They walked single file, the larger European first, followed by a Chinese who was using the European as a shield against the driving wind.

Neither had experienced such weather before. The Taiwanese doctor had just arrived in Omaha to begin a 1 year esophageal research fellowship. The Italian doctor had started his fellowship at the University of Chicago and volunteered to help me move to Creighton University in Omaha. At Creighton University he would continue his esophageal research fellow and together we would set up the esophageal motility laboratory, reinitiate the studies we had ongoing at the University of Chicago, and start an esophageal surgical practice in mid-America. His name was Dr. Luigi Bonavina. He came highly recommended by his Professor, Alberto Peracchia, then the chairman of the Department of Surgery at the University of Padua. Little did I know that a lifelong friendship was kindling and over time this student would become my mentor.

The first study we did together was on pharyngo-esophageal dysfunction and was presented in Colorado Springs, Colorado, to the Western Surgical Association on November 12, 1984. Based on the number of citations, the most popular manuscript we wrote during his fellowship was published in *Annals of Surgery* in 1986 and entitled "Nissen Fundoplication for Gastroesophageal Reflux Disease: Evaluation of Primary Repair in 100 Consecutive Patients." The experience Dr. Bonavina gained in putting this manuscript together served as a template for the subsequent contributions he has made over the years.

It is now over a quarter of a century later and Professor Bonavina has become a leader in the European world of esophageal surgery with a reputation that extends around the globe. Over the years he has developed a keen understanding of esophageal physiology. He is a careful surgeon, experienced in minimally invasive procedures and gifted with exquisite surgical skill. It was an easy choice for Mr. Todd Berg, the chief executive officer of Torax Medical, Inc. and developer of an innovative anti-reflux device, to select Professor Bonavina's unit to initiate the European arm of a feasibility clinical trial. In his typical workable manner, Professor Bonavina graciously took on the task. Now, with three peer review publications on the subject and soon to have implanted over 100 LINX devices, Professor Bonavina has put his reputation behind the innovation.

These efforts have sparked the creation of the book you have before you. For surgery to move from the reputation of a therapy of last resort for esophageal disease to a therapy for the early stages of esophageal disease requires two conditions: first, an understanding of the pathophysiologic abnormality of the disease and second the availability of a simplified,safe and effective outpatient surgical procedure that dependably corrects the dysfunction. Clinical investigators have been occupied with the simplification of existing and the introduction of new, unique and less invasive procedures to treat a variety of esophageal conditions since the turn of the century. I am pleased Professor Bonavina had the vision and energy to organize a meeting of esophageal clinical scientists from throughout the world and publish a book to follow on the subject of "Innovation in Esophageal Surgery". No one is more suited to have done it!

Department of Surgery
University of Southern California

Tom R. DeMeester, M.D.

Preface

Over the past decade there has been an impressive evolution in the field of esophageal surgery. Significant advancements in diagnostics and technical refinements of complex minimally invasive procedures have indeed driven this surgical specialty to high levels of excellence. The concept of a multidisciplinary approach to esophageal disease has now been accepted by most physicians, and with the tremendous increase in the incidence of esophageal adenocarcinoma, the need for a more focused postgraduate training in foregut surgery has emerged.

In November 2011, an international meeting entitled "Innovation in Esophageal Surgery" was organized in Milan to celebrate the 10th year of activity of the Center for Esophageal Disease at IRCCS Policlinico San Donato, one of the main teaching hospitals of the University of Milan Medical School. This was also a great occasion to celebrate the 80th birthday of Professor Alberto Peracchia, my "master" of surgery, a true pioneer and innovator in esophageal surgery when this discipline was still neglected by many. He has been a unique teacher and mentor, a superb surgeon, a great innovator, and a truly international leader.

I was able to gather in San Donato a distinguished faculty from 13 countries to share science and experience with centers of excellence worldwide. I am very grateful to all speakers who accepted to participate in this unique event and to those who agreed to contribute to this volume. I am deeply indebted to Tom DeMeester, unique mentor, pioneer, great innovator, and leader in esophagology. He has been very influential in my surgical career, a true icon and a great source of inspiration. I am also very grateful to Giuseppe Rotelli, President of the Gruppo San Donato, who trusted me since the beginning of my activity at Policlinico San Donato and honored me with his friendship and encouragement. His continuous support has contributed so much to the quality of care delivered by my team to all patients referred to the Center for Esophageal Disease.

This book introduces the general and the thoracic surgeon to the latest developments in esophageal surgery. In each chapter the reader will find an updated state-of-the-art review of innovative methods and techniques which have had a significant impact on clinical practice over the past decade. Despite the tremendous pressure to reduce cost of health care and despite resistance to change by part of the medical and surgical community, innovation remains a powerful engine for human progress. I hope that *Innovation in Esophageal Surgery* will be highly informative for both the novice and the expert surgeon wishing to enter the intriguing arena of esophageal surgery.

Luigi Bonavina

Acknowledgments

I would like to express my gratitude to all teachers, mentors, partners, trainees, and medical students who have inspired my professional career. A special tribute to the memory of my father Francesco Bonavina, my first teacher and mentor of humanities and medicine. Last but not least, thanks to the women of my life, Elisabetta, Giulia, and Francesca, for their understanding, tolerance, and continuing support.

Contents

Contributors

Surya S.A.Y. Biere Department of Surgery, VU University Medical Centre, Amsterdam, The Netherlands

Davide Bona Department of Biomedical Sciences for Health, Division of General Surgery, IRCCS Policlinico San Donato, University of Milano School of Medicine, San Donato Milanese (Milan), Italy

Luigi Bonavina Department of Biomedical Sciences for Health, Division of General Surgery, IRCCS Policlinico San Donato, University of Milan School of Medicine, San Donato Milanese (Milan), Italy

Marco Braga Department of Surgery, San Raffaele University, Milan, Italy

Wolfram Breithaupt Department of General-, Visceral- and Thoracic Surgery, AGAPLESION Markus Krankenhaus, Frankfurt am Main, Germany

Miguel A. Cuesta Department of Surgery, VU University Medical Centre, Amsterdam, The Netherlands

Tom R. DeMeester Department of Surgery, Keck School of Medicine, University of Southern California, Los Angeles, CA, USA

Steven R. DeMeester Department of Surgery, Keck School of Medicine, University of Southern California, Los Angeles, CA, USA

Ulrich K. Fetzner Department of General, Visceral and Cancer Surgery, University of Cologne, Cologne, Germany

Karl-Hermann Fuchs Department of General-, Visceral- and Thoracic Surgery, AGAPLESION Markus Krankenhaus, Frankfurt am Main, Germany

Suzanne S. Gisbertz Department of Surgery, VU University Medical Centre, Amsterdam, The Netherlands

S. Michael Griffin Northern Oesophago-Gastric Cancer Unit, Royal Victoria Infirmary, Newcastle upon Tyne, UK

Marion Hädrich Division of Gastroenteroiogy, University Clinic for Visceral Surgery and Medicine, Bern University Hospital, Bern, Switzerland

Arnulf H. Hölscher Department of General, Visceral and Cancer Surgery, University of Cologne, Cologne, Germany

Mark D. Iannettoni Department of Cardiothoracic Surgery, University of Iowa Hospitals and Clinics, Iowa City, IA, USA

Simon Law Department of Surgery, Division of Esophageal and Upper Gastrointestinal Surgery, The University of Hong Kong, Queen Mary Hospital, Hong Kong, China

Emanuele Meroni Department of Diagnostic Endoscopy and Endoscopic Surgery, Istituto Nazionale Tumori, Milan, Italy

Jeffrey H. Peters Division of Thoracic and Foregut Surgery, Department of Surgery, University of Rochester School of Medicine and Dentistry, Rochester, NY, USA

Francesca Rancati Medical Affairs Department, Bârrx Medical, Inc, Malnate (VA), Italy

Martin Riegler University Clinic of Surgery, Medical University Vienna, Vienna General Hospital, Vienna, Austria

Greta Saino Department of Biomedical Sciences for Health, Division of General Surgery, IRCCS Policlinico San Donato, University of Milano School of Medicine, San Donato Milanese (Milan), Italy

Sebastian F. Schoppmann Department of General Surgery, University Clinic of Surgery, Medical University Vienna, Vienna, Austria

Stephanie Fischer See Manometry Lab, University Clinic of Surgery, Medical University Vienna, Vienna, Austria

Joel Shapiro Department of Surgery, Erasmus Medical Center, Rotterdam, Zuid-Holland, The Netherlands

Radu Tutuian Division of Gastroenterology, University Clinic for Visceral Surgery and Medicine, Bern University Hospital, Bern, Switzerland

Mark van Berge Henegouwen Department of Surgery, Academic Medical Centre, Amsterdam, The Netherlands

J. Jan B. van Lanschot Department of Surgery, Erasmus Medical Center, Rotterdam, Zuid-Holland, The Netherlands

Donald L. van der Peet Department of Surgery, VU University Medical Centre, Amsterdam, The Netherlands

Gábor Varga Department of General-, Visceral- and Thoracic Surgery, AGAPLESION Markus Krankenhaus, Frankfurt am Main, Germany

Daniel von Renteln Department of Endoscopy, University Hospital Hamburg Eppendorf, Martinistrasse, Hamburg, Germany

Shajahan Wahed Northern Oesophago-Gastric Cancer Unit, Royal Victoria Infirmary, Newcastle upon Tyne, UK

Thomas J. Watson Division of Thoracic and Foregut Surgery, Department of Surgery, University of Rochester School of Medicine and Dentistry, Rochester, NY, USA

Johannes Zacherl Department of General Surgery, University Clinic of Surgery, Medical University Vienna, Vienna, Austria

Assessment of Surgical Innovation

1

Luigi Bonavina

...imagination is more important than knowledge (Albert Einstein)
...stay hungry, stay foolish (Steve Jobs)
...primum non nocere (Hippocrates)

In general, progress in surgery depends on experience in the care of patients, accurate record keeping, reflection on the experience, structuring of subsequent clinical experience, and, finally, honest and effective reporting of the results to the surgical community. Often, it takes years before new concepts are accepted, and there are many examples of how the best innovations are greeted with envy and skepticism [1]. In 1805, the first effective lighting system for endoscopy invented by Philippe Bozzini was rejected by the medical faculty of Vienna which defined the new discovery as the "magic lantern" [2].

The Society for University Surgeons Surgical Innovations Project Team described innovation as "… *a new or modified surgical procedure that differs from currently accepted local practice, the outcomes of which have not been described, and which may entail risk to the patient*" [3]. Often, in the surgical world, the rationale for adopting innovative techniques or technologies is not evidence-based, and the assessment of surgical innovation is a complex task. This fact applies also to esophageal surgery, which is unanimously recognized as a highly challenging discipline due to the difficulties in interpreting pathophysiology, standardizing surgical technique, tailoring the operation to the individual patient, reducing postoperative morbidity, and improving patient's quality of life. As a consequence, adoption of innovative procedures in this specialty is usually restricted to a few centers of excellence where the experience of individual surgeons influences the outcome and is an independent factor of quality of hospital care. Still, high-quality evidence coming from large, multicenter and randomized studies is lacking [4, 5].

On the other hand, it should be admitted that a randomized trial is not always required to change existing surgical paradigms. The old dogma assuming that a "big surgeon makes big incisions" is no longer compatible with modern surgical practice. Laparoscopic cholecystectomy, first performed in 1987 by Philippe Mouret, was not initially evaluated by randomized clinical trials but emerged by case series as a "disruptive" innovation [6]. As Atul Gawande pointed out in his recent review of 200 years of surgery, "*Minimization of the invasiveness of surgical procedures is an advance that is arguably as significant as the discovery of anesthesia*" [7].

Today, the advent of Natural Orifice Transluminal Endoscopic Surgery (NOTES) exemplifies a *déjà-vu* phenomenon, the gap that separates the innovators from the majority of practicing surgeons. NOTES has evolved from experimental work [8], and the feasibility of intraluminal surgical interventions with access through the transesophageal, transgastric, transrectal, transvescical and transvaginal routes, and

L. Bonavina
Department of Biomedical Sciences for Health,
Division of General Surgery,
IRCCS Policlinico San Donato,
University of Milan School of Medicine,
Piazza Malan 2, 20097
San Donato Milanese (Milan), Italy
e-mail: luigi.bonavina@unimi.it

L. Bonavina (ed.), *Innovation in Esophageal Surgery*,
DOI 10.1007/978-88-470-2469-4_1, © Springer-Verlag Italia 2012

without the need for skin incisions, has been demonstrated. However, it is not straightforward for a new technology to go through all stages of development: it must prove better, faster, safer, more cosmetically attractive, and cheaper, but advancement in these categories is not an "all-or-nothing" event. Gains made in some areas may be offset by losses in other areas, still the net gain must be enough to bridge the gap.

Despite the current trend toward reduction of health-care costs and the strenuous resistance to change by some professional and academic authorities, innovation is regarded today as the vital lymph and the only long-term solution to high-quality, affordable health care [9]. It is critical, however, to improve the pathway of surgical innovation so that decisions can be based on high-quality outcome data. The Balliol Colloquia first introduced a framework to safely and effectively translate surgical innovations into clinical practice [10–12]. The acronym IDEAL (Idea, Development, Evaluation, Assessment, Long-term study) was proposed to define the crucial steps that should be followed to provide reporting of implementation and adoption of new surgical techniques. It has recently been shown that the IDEAL framework is a feasible method to document the implementation and development of minimally invasive esophagectomy [13]. Talking to patients about innovative surgical procedures could effectively supplement the IDEAL framework, since the actual number of patients being offered, accepting, and declining a new procedure should always be reported [14].

Responsible surgical innovation is needed in the present era of cost-containment, increased complexity in ethical issues, and deterioration of the patient-physician relationship. Since it is impossible to design implantable medical devices with zero risk of failure, post-marketing surveillance is very critical to assure long-term safety. Clinical registries operated by independent professional organizations are clearly necessary to protect the public health from the risks inherent in the innovations [15, 16].

Surgical innovation has become a complex process that needs to be properly regulated before widespread clinical application. Enthusiasm for innovation should always be balanced by concern for patient's safety and well-being. Surgical research, supported by human creativity, intuition, resilience, and serendipity, will move forward the legacy of the great pioneers of the past by promoting innovation and by improving patient care.

Key Points

- Innovation is vital lymph in surgery
- Intuition and creativity play a major role in the early stage of the process
- Development and application of surgical innovations require high-quality outcome data
- Clinical registries and post-marketing surveillance of implantable devices are critical to ensure patient safety

References

1. Lillehei W (1995) New ideas and their acceptance. As it has related to preservation of chordae tendinea and certain other discoveries. J Heart Valve Dis 4(suppl 2): S106–S114
2. Gorden A (1993) The history and development of endoscopic surgery. Saunders, London
3. Biffl WL, Spain DA, Reitsma AM et al (2008) Responsible development and application of surgical innovations: a position statement of the Society of University Surgeons. J Am Coll Surg 206:1204–1209
4. Bone J, Livestro DP, Elias SG, Borel Rinkes IHM, van Hillegersberg R (2009) International survey on esophageal cancer: part I surgical techniques. Dis Esophagus 22:195–202
5. Lagarde SM, Vrouenraets BC, Stassen LPS, Van Lanschot JJB (2010) Evidence-based surgical treatment of esophageal cancer: overview of high-quality studies. Ann Thorac Surg 89:1319–1326
6. Riskin DJ, Longaker MT, Gertner M, Krummel TM (2006) Innovation in surgery. A historical perspective. Ann Surg 244:686–693
7. Gawande A (2012) Two hundred years of surgery. N Engl J Med 366:1716–1723
8. Kalloo AN, Singh VK, Jagannath SB et al (2004) Flexible transgastric peritoneoscopy: a novel approach to diagnostic and therapeutic interventions. Gastrointest Endosc 60:114–117
9. Cosgrove DM (2000) The innovation imperative. J Thorac Cardiovasc Surg 120:839–842

10. Barkun JS, Aronson JK, Feldman LS, Maddern GJ, Strasberg SM, for the Balliol Collaboration (2009) Evaluation and stages of surgical innovations. Lancet 374:1089–1096
11. Ergina PL, Cook JA, Blazeby JM et al (2009) Challenges in evaluating surgical innovation. Lancet 374:1097–1104
12. McCulloch P, Altman DG, Campbell WB et al (2009) No surgical innovation without evaluation: the IDEAL recommendations. Lancet 374:1105–1112
13. Blazeby JM, Blencowe NS, Titcomb DR, Metcalfe C, Hollowood AD, Barham CP (2011) Demonstration of the IDEAL recommendations for evaluating and reporting surgical innovation in minimally invasive oesophagectomy. Br J Surg 98:544–551
14. Blazeby JM, McNair AGK (2011) Commentary: talking to patients about surgical innovations. BMJ 342:d2871
15. Avorn J (2010) Regulation of devices. BMJ 341:c5730
16. Resnic FS, Normand SLT (2012) Postmarketing surveillance of medical devices – filling in the gaps. N Engl J Med 366(10):875–877

2 Clinical Impact of High-Resolution Manometry and Impedance-pH Monitoring

Marion Hädrich and Radu Tutuian

2.1 Introduction

Deglutition is an important physiologic process ensuring our ability to ingest food and liquids. Under normal conditions we swallow approximately 600–2,500 times a day without effort or even noticing the complexity of this process [1]. After the oral and pharyngeal phase of deglutition the bolus is transported through the esophagus into the stomach by involuntary neuromuscular reflexes (i.e. the process of esophageal peristalsis) followed by the relaxation of the lower esophageal sphincter. Impaired swallowing (i.e. dysphagia) causes discomfort and limits our daily activity. Patients with esophageal symptoms (such as dysphagia and/or retrosternal chest pain) seeking medical attention should be referred to gastrointestinal (GI) specialists for detailed investigations. After having excluded structural lesions by endoscopy or barium esophagogram patients should undergo esophageal function testing to investigate esophageal motility abnormalities as a cause of their symptoms.

Heartburn and regurgitation are typical gastroesophageal reflux disease (GERD) symptoms. Current estimates suggest that approximate 40 % of the adult US population experience these symptoms at least once a week, making GERD the most common reason for outpatient GI consultation [2]. Patients with GERD symptoms are often treated with proton pump inhibitors (PPIs) by primary care physicians and those with severe, alarm or persistent symptoms are referred for further testing to GI specialists. An upper GI endoscopy performed to evaluate esophageal erosions as the hallmark of GERD finds erosive esophagitis in only 30 % of patients [3]. Patients with esophageal symptoms and normal esophageal mucosa are referred for esophageal reflux monitoring in order to assess esophageal acid exposure and the relationship between symptoms and gastroesophageal reflux episodes.

Over the years esophageal manometry and pH-monitoring have come to be regarded as the gold standards for testing esophageal motility and quantifying gastroesophageal reflux respectively. Recent technical and computational developments now make it possible to generate detailed pressure maps of the esophagus using high-resolution manometry and to detect gastroesophageal reflux independently of its acidic contents using impedance-pH monitoring. In the present chapter we review the use of high-resolution manometry (HRM) and multichannel intraluminal impedance-pH (MII-pH) monitoring in clinical practice.

M. Hädrich • R. Tutuian (✉)
Division of Gastroenterology, University Clinic for Visceral Surgery and Medicine,
Bern University Hospital, Bern 3010, Switzerland
e-mail: marion.haedrich@insel.ch; radu.tutian@insel.ch

L. Bonavina (ed.), *Innovation in Esophageal Surgery*,
DOI 10.1007/978-88-470-2469-4_2, © Springer-Verlag Italia 2012

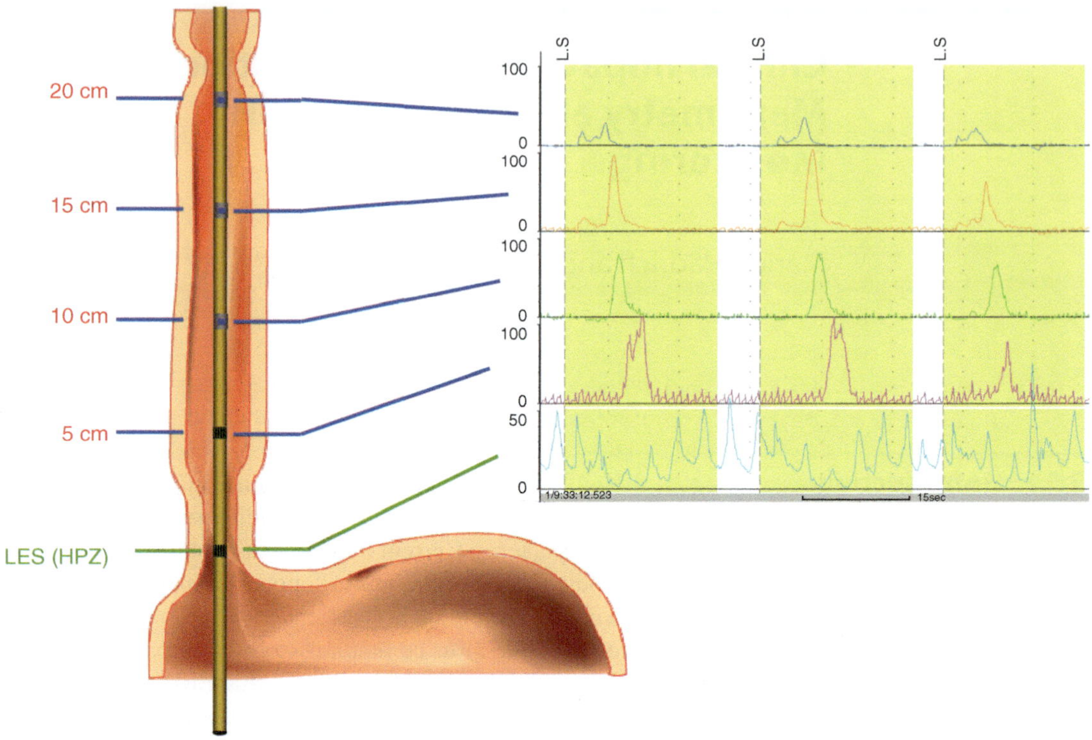

Fig. 2.1 Conventional esophageal manometry using five pressure sensors located in the lower esophageal sphincter (*LES*) high pressure zone (*HPZ*) and esophageal body 5, 10, 15 and 20 cm above the LES

2.2 Esophageal Motility Testing Using High-Resolution Manometry

Esophageal manometry is used in clinical practice to quantify contraction amplitude, peristaltic velocity and sphincter relaxation (both upper and lower esophageal sphincter) during deglutition. Manometry systems consist of a catheter with built-in (solid state) or external pressure transducers (pressure being transmitted from esophagus to sensor by water-perfused catheter), a pressure recorder and a computer with dedicated software for analysis. Esophageal manometry is performed under local anesthesia after the patient has fasted for 4–6 h. The probe is inserted and after localizing the lower esophageal sphincter (LES) and measuring the resting pressure of the LES 10 swallows are performed 20–30 s apart in order to prevent deglutitive inhibition.

In conventional manometry it is possible to analyze the upper esophageal sphincter pressure, the contraction amplitude duration and contraction onset velocity. In conventional esophageal manometry normal peristalsis is achieved if the contraction amplitude exceeds 30 mmHg at two pressure sites in the distal esophagus spaced 5 cm apart and if the contraction onset velocity between these two sites is less than 8 cm/s. A contraction amplitude below 30 mmHg at one site is considered an ineffective contraction and a contraction onset velocity more than 8 cm/s between the (5-cm apart) sites is considered a simultaneous contraction if the contraction amplitude exceeds 30 mmHg. The normal value of the lower esophageal sphincter ranges from 10 to 45 mmHg with a residual pressure <8 mmHg in conventional esophageal manometry [4] (Fig. 2.1).

Since the introduction of esophageal manometry into clinical practice more than 50 years ago important developments have taken place. Recent developments include high-resolution manometry and high-resolution impedance manometry. High-resolution manometry (HRM) uses closely spaced pressure sensors (usually 1–1.5 cm apart) with 20–36 channels per catheter. The software interpolates values between sensors providing a virtually continuous pressure map of the esophagus and its sphincters. The line plots are replaced by esophageal pressure topography graphs with time on the x-axis, distance of the pressure sensors from the nose on the y-axis and pressure magnitude on the z-axis, scaled by colour intensity. In the colour contour plot isobaric contours are displayed as a continuous line of a value of equal pressure on a pressure topography plot (Fig. 2.2). HRM visualizes the pressure topography of the esophagus in a way that is easy to understand (even for non-professionals after a short training), reliable and reproducible [5]. By the two-dimensional picturing of the measurements it is simple to identify normal contractions, primary vs. secondary peristalsis, hiatal hernias and the contractile features of the esophagus and even other high-pressure zones (i.e. an accentuated aortic arch or an augmented left atrium).

The field of applications ranges from the investigation of non-cardiac chest pain and of non obstructive dysphagia, preoperative evaluations before bariatric or anti-reflux surgery and in advance of an impedance-pH manometry with a view to localizing the lower esophageal sphincter for the positioning of the MII-pH impedance probe.

In the characterization of the esophago-gastric junction (EGJ) pressure morphology it is important to remember the components of the pressure profile of the EGJ: the lower esophageal sphincter (LES) and the crural diaphragm (CD). In the case of a hiatal hernia with a double-pressure zone the fixed high-pressure zone independent of the respiration can be identified as the LES, and the high-pressure zone changing with respiration as the CD. The respiratory inversion point is the junction between intra-abdominal and intra-mediastinal pressure, defined as the position where the inspiratory EGJ pressure becomes less than the expiratory EGJ pressure. EGJ relaxation is measured in the deglutitive relaxation window, starting with the upper esophageal sphincter (UES) relaxation until the arrival of the peristaltic contraction arrives at the EGJ. Ghosh et al. proposed in 2007 after a quantitative analysis of 400 patients and 75 controls the integrated relaxation pressure computed over 4 s (IRP-4 s) as a parameter to quantify deglutitive LES relaxation [6].

The report of the analysis of the distal segment contractility contains the peristalsis, which is composed of a proximal segment with striated muscles and a distal segment with another three sub-segments with smooth muscles, interadjacent the transition zone. Contractile front velocity (CFV) measures the velocity of the conduction of the peristaltic contraction in cm/s at the isobaric contour of 30 mmHg beginning at the transition zone until the proximal EGJ with values up to 8.5 cm/s as the norm. The distal contractile integral (DCI) quantifies the esophageal peristalsis by integrating pressure, duration and distance of the peristaltic wave in the distal esophagus. Normal DCI values are below 5,000 mmHg · s · cm (Table 2.1).

The technical developments of HRM were followed by a revised classification of motility abnormalities. The Chicago classification integrates the morphology and pressure characteristics of the EGJ, EGJ relaxation, CFV and DCI of the peristalsis so making it possible to classify nutcracker esophagus subtypes, esophageal spasm and three subtypes of achalasia [7, 8] (Fig. 2.3). At first the EGJ has to be characterized by morphology and deglutitive EGJ relaxation (normal integrated relaxation pressure (IRP) < 15 mmHg). In the case of normal deglutitive EGJ relaxation an isobaric contour at 30 mmHg is drawn and the integrity of this isobaric area analyzed. In patients with continuous isobaric 30 mmHg contour the DCI is used to define hypertensive contractions (DCI > 5,000 mmHg · s · cm; nutcracker esophagus) or hypercontractile esophagus (DCI > 8,000 mmHg · s · cm; jackhammer esophagus) or normal esophageal peristalsis. In the case of breaks in the isobaric 30 mmHg contour Bulsiewicz et al. proposed a division into large (>2 cm) or small (<2 cm) breaks, the first

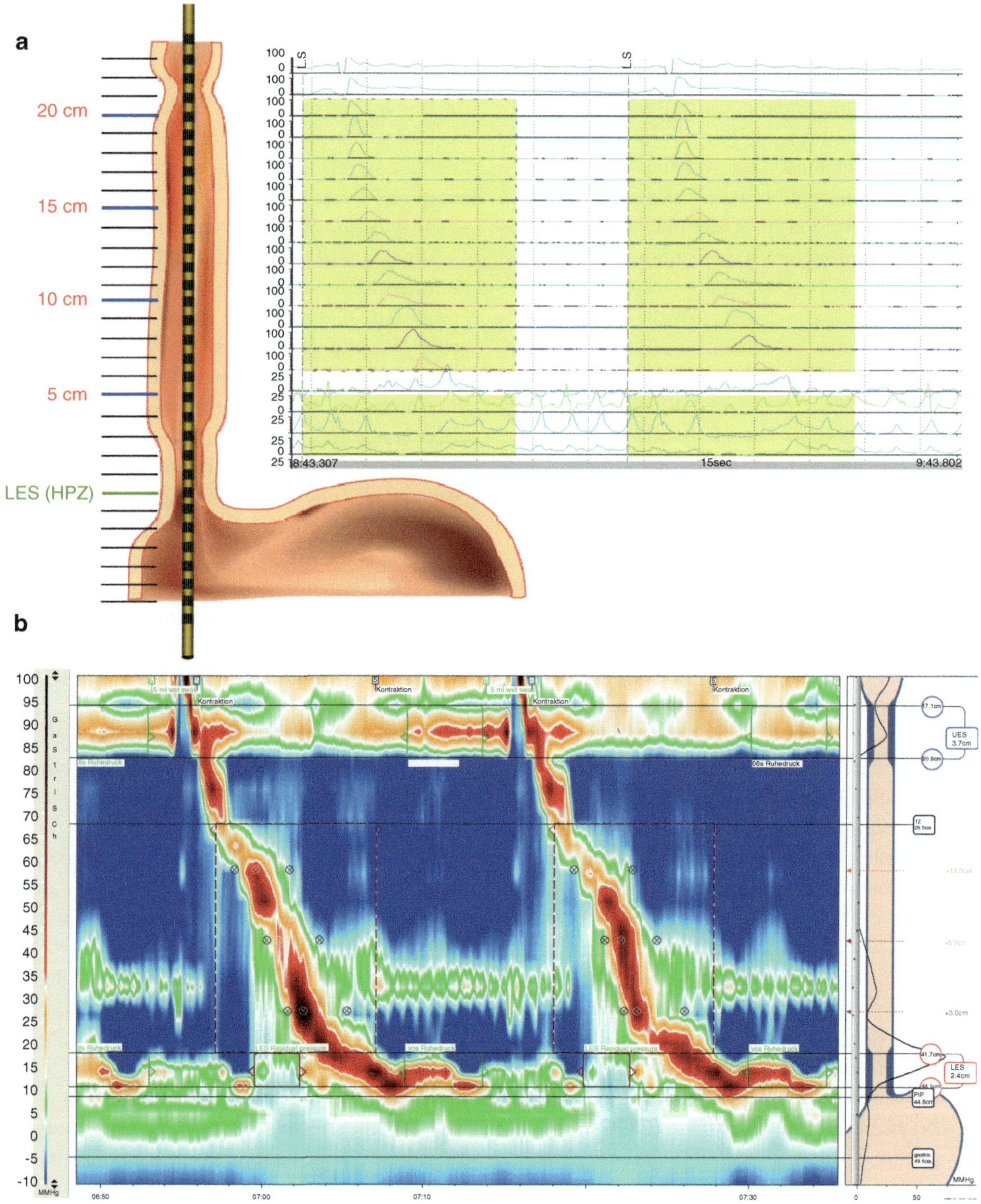

Fig. 2.2 High-resolution esophageal manometry. Esophageal pressure data is collected from sensors placed at a distance of 1–1.5 cm from each other (**a**). In pressure topography the pharyngeal contraction, upper esophageal sphincter relaxation (normal 300–500 ms), proximal esophageal peristalsis, transition zone (*TZ*), distal esophageal peristalsis and lower esophageal sphincter (*LES*) relaxation (normal 6–10 s) can be quantified for each swallow (**b**)

Table 2.1 High resolution manometry (HRM) diagnostic criteria for esophageal motility abnormalities

Normal	
	Defect in the 30 mmHg isobaric contour in the distal segment of the esophagus <3 cm
	CFV < 8 cm s^{-1} in >90 % of swallows, IBP < 15 mmHg, DCI < 5,000 mmHg · s · cm
	Normal EGJ relaxation (mean IRP < 15 mmHg) and normal IBP (10–35 mmHg)
Hypotensive peristalsis	
	>3 cm defects in the 30 mmHg isobaric contour of the distal esophageal segment
	Intermittent: > 30 % swallows with hypotensive or absent peristalsis
	Frequent: > 70 % swallows with hypotensive or absent peristalsis
Absent peristalsis	
	No propagating contractile wavefront in 100 % of swallows
	No isobaric pressurization greater than 30 mmHg isobaric contour
Hypertensive peristalsis	
	Normal peristaltic velocity <8 cm/s in >80 % of swallows
	Mean DCI > 5,000 mmHg · s · cm or LES after contraction >180 mmHg
	Normal CVF
Spastic nutcracker	
	Normal CVF, Mean DCI > 8,000 mmHg · s · cm
Esophageal spasm (rapidly propagated contractile wavefront)	
	Spasm (CVF > 8 cm s^{-1}) in >20 % of swallows
	Segmental spasm: Spasm limited to one of the three segments of the distal esophagus
	Diffuse spasm: Spasm involving both upper segments of the distal esophagus
Peristaltic dysfunction	
	Mild: 3–6 swallows with failed peristalsis or a >2 cm defect in the 30 mmHg isobaric contour of the distal esophageal peristalsis
	Severe: ≥7 swallows with either failed peristalsis or a >2 cm defect in the 30 mmHg isobaric contour of distal esophageal peristalsis
	Aperistalsis: Contractile pressure <30 mmHg throughout mid-distal esophagus in all swallows (Scleroderma pattern: aperistalsis with LES pressure <10 mmHg)
Achalasia	
	Impaired deglutitive EGJ relaxation and/or opening
	Elevation of intra-esophageal bolus pressure due to resistance to flow at EGJ
	Classic: Mean IRP > 15 mmHg, aperistalsis
	Achalasia with compression: Mean IRP > 15 mmHg, absent peristalsis with compartmentalized pressurizations
	Spastic achalasia: Mean IRP > 15 mmHg, absent peristalsis and spasms (CFV > 8 cm s^{-1})
Abnormal LES tone	
	Hypotensive: 10 s mean < 10 mmHg with normal peristaltic function
	Hypertensive: 10 s mean > 35 mmHg with normal peristaltic function and EGJ relaxation

Adapted from [8]

CFV contractile front velocity, *DCI* distal contractile index, *EGJ* esophago-gastric junction, *IBP* Intrabolus pressure, *IRP* integrated relaxation pressure, *LES* lower esophageal sphincter

ones being more often associated with impaired esophageal bolus clearance [9].

2.2.1 Achalasia

Achalasia is a primary esophageal motor disease caused by destruction of the inhibitory neurons in the Auerbach plexus of the entire esophagus resulting in a complete lack of peristalsis. It causes often dysphagia, regurgitation with risk of aspiration, chest pain and in the course of the disease weight loss. It is defined as aperistalsis and impaired deglutitive EGJ relaxation.

High-resolution manometry (HRM) brought novel criteria and sub-classification criteria for achalasia. Pandolfino et al. found that an elevated integrated residual pressure (IRP) > 15 mmHg in the absence of esophageal peristalsis had a sensitivity of 98 % and a specificity of 96 % to diagnose achalasia [10]. With HRM the sensitivity of the detection of achalasia improved, but more important a new classification of clinically relevant subtypes of achalasia was developed. Classic type I achalasia includes patients with elevated IRP and absent esophageal peristalsis. Type II achalasia (with pressurization) is characterized by elevated IRP and absent peristalsis but elevated

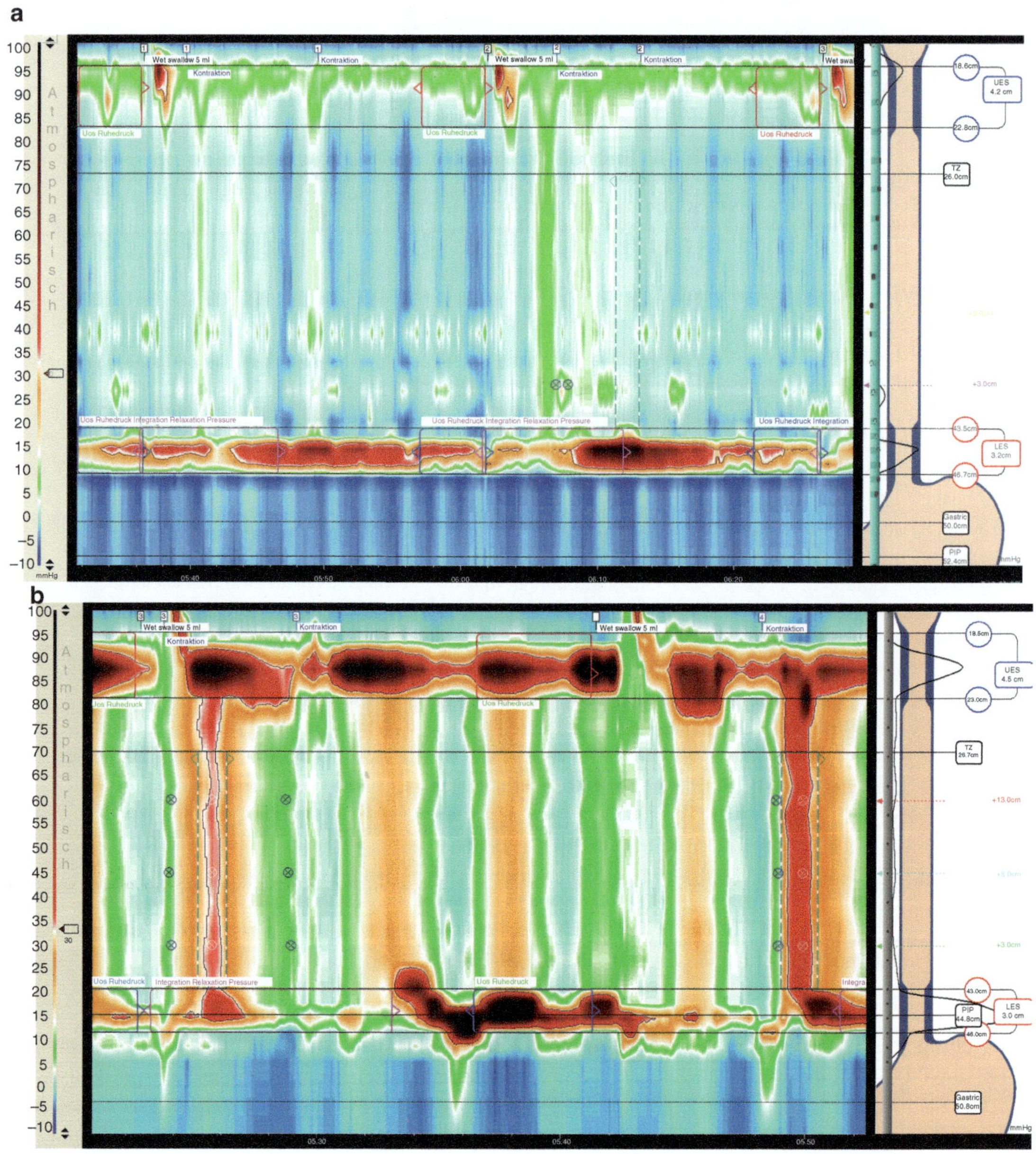

Fig. 2.3 Subtypes of achalasia: (**a**) type I classic achalasia – impaired EGJ relaxation and absent esophageal peristalsis; (**b**) type II with pressurization – impaired EGJ relaxation and non-peristaltic pressure changes exceeding 30 mmHg; (**c**) type III with spasms – more than 80 % spastic contractions in the distal esophagus with impaired EGJ relaxation. *EGJ* esophago-gastric junction

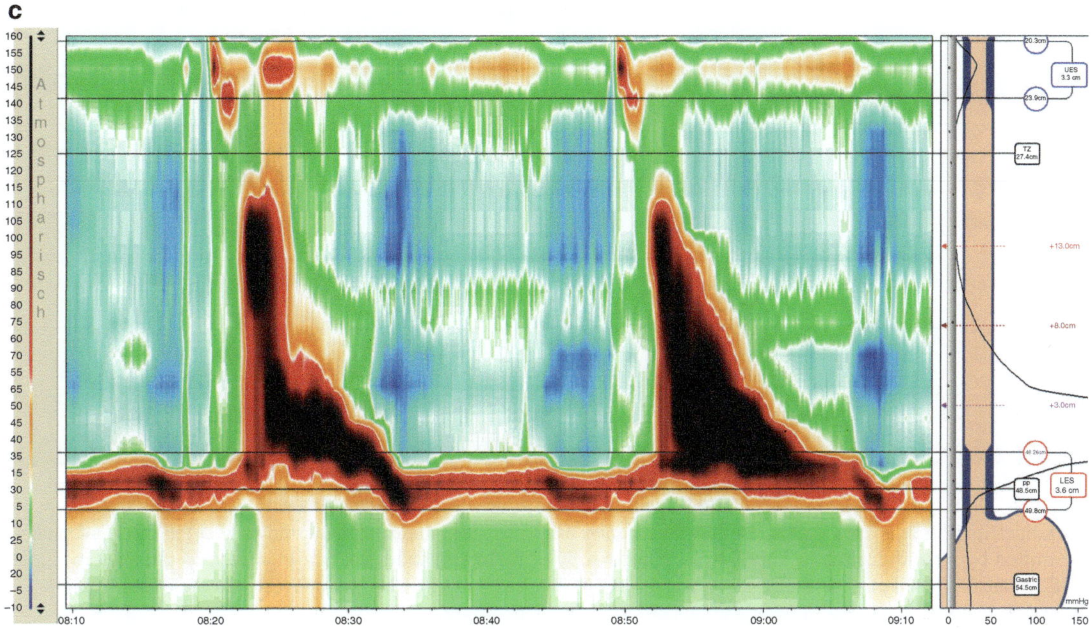

Fig. 2.3 (continued)

panesophageal pressure (>30 mmHg). This corresponds to the previously defined *vigorous achalasia* by Spechler and Castell. Achalasia with compression shows a panesophageal pressurization and has the best outcome with a positive treatment response of 100 % to Heller myotomy and 91 % to pneumatic dilatation reported in 49 newly diagnosed type II achalasia patients. The least frequent pattern is type III achalasia (with spasms) characterized by impaired EGJ relaxation (i.e. elevated IRP) and with spastic contraction in the distal esophagus. Outcome studies suggest that this type (type III achalasia) has the overall poorest response to therapy (29 % overall).

2.3 Gastroesophageal Reflux Testing Using Combined Impedance-pH Monitoring

With each deglutition during meals we ingest small amounts of air that accumulate in the stomach and are subsequently released by belching. This process involves reflex, transient relaxations of the lower esophageal sphincter (tLESRs) induced by distension of gastric fundus. Depending on the filling of the stomach, occasionally small amounts of liquids (or mixture of liquid and gas) can reflux back from the stomach into the esophagus. As long as these episodes (in normal individuals up to 50 episodes per day) are not associated with symptoms or do not cause esophageal lesions by prolonged esophageal acid exposure gastroesophageal reflux remains undetected. Increased body fat (i.e. increased body mass index), large/cal-rich meals and modern lifestyle (with large evening meals within a couple of hours of going to bed) are some of the factors that lead to an increased prevalence of gastroesophageal disease (GERD). In the mid 1980s potent acid suppressive therapy using proton pump inhibitors (PPIs) provided important relief for a disease that affects 15–20 % of the adult population. Therapy with PPIs had an important impact not only on the natural course and therapy of GERD but also brought new challenges for the diagnosis of GERD.

Esophageal pH-monitoring uses the low pH of the gastric content to identify gastroesophageal reflux episodes. This method, introduced in the early 1970s, soon became the gold standard to diagnose GERD, in particular in patients with

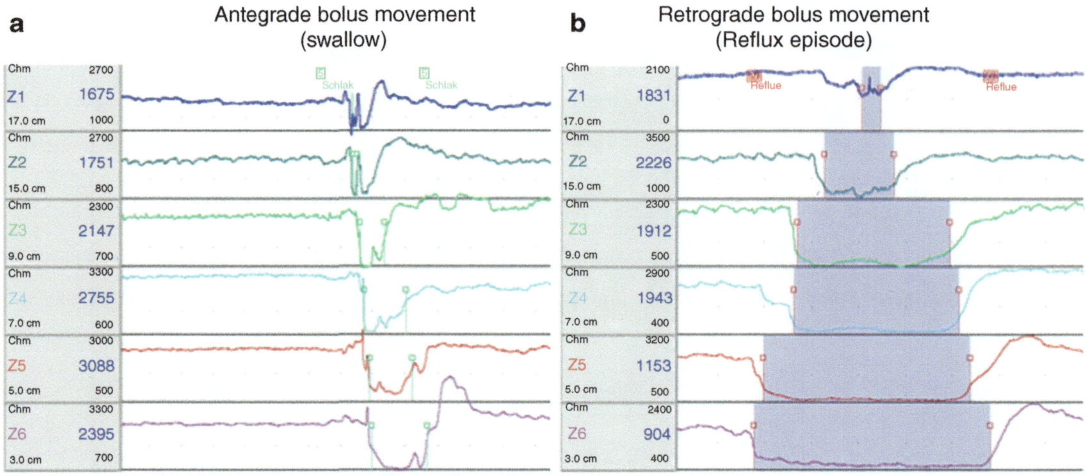

Fig. 2.4 Bolus presence and movement detected by multichannel intraluminal impedance. Liquid bolus entry is identified by a rapid decline in impedance, bolus exit by the return of impedance to baseline. Serial impedance measurement segments on a catheter can be used to determine the direction of bolus movement: swallows (**a**) are characterized by declines in impedance starting in the proximal and over time moving to the distal esophagus. Reflux episodes (**b**) are identified as declines in impedance starting distally and over time moving to the proximal esophagus

normal esophageal mucosa. Quantifying gastroesophageal reflux by monitoring intraluminal pH becomes difficult if gastric acidity is suppressed by PPIs, a common first-line scenario used for patients with typical (heartburn and/or regurgitation) and atypical (chest pain, hoarseness, epigastric burning, etc.) GERD symptoms. Among several methods attempting to overcome these limitations, multichannel intraluminal impedance monitoring has become the method of choice to identify gastroesophageal reflux episodes.

Multichannel intraluminal impedance (MII) measures resistance to an alternating electrical current between two electrodes placed within the esophageal lumen. In an empty esophagus the electrical circuit is closed by the esophageal mucosa that provides a resistance of 1,500–2,000 Ω. Liquids arriving in an impedance-measuring segment produce a rapid decline in impedance by improving electrical conductivity through the ionic charges within the bolus. Lining up multiple impedance measuring segments along a catheter allows to detect not only bolus presence but also the direction of bolus movement. Changes in intraluminal impedance progressing over time from proximal to distal indicate an aboral, antegrade bolus movement as seen during swallowing while changes progressing over time from distal to proximal indicate an oral, retrograde bolus movement as seen during reflux episodes (Fig. 2.4). Furthermore impedance measurements provide information on the physical properties of the refluxate. Pure liquid reflux episodes produce only declines in impedance (progressing from distal to proximal) while pure gas reflux episodes (belching) produce only a rise in impedance. The combination of increases and declines in intraluminal impedance indicate mixed (liquid–gas or gas–liquid) content of the refluxate. Combining MII with pH (MII-pH) makes it possible to detect reflux episodes of all types and classify them into acid or non-acid by their nadir pH (acid – nadir pH < 4; non-acid – nadir pH > 4).

Over the years MII-pH data recorded in healthy volunteers have served as a basis for establishing normal values. Two multicenter studies from US-Belgian [11] and French-Belgian [12] groups provided normal values for the total number of reflux episodes (acid and non-acid, liquid and mixed), proximal extent of reflux episodes and esophageal acid exposure off PPI therapy. A subsequent study by Zentilin et al. provided

Table 2.2 Normal values for combined MII-pH monitoring based on 95th percentile data in healthy volunteers not taking acid suppressive therapy

		Impedance-pH monitoring		
		US-Belgian (N = 60)	French-Belgian (N = 72)	Italian (N = 25)
Esophageal pH data				
% time pH <4	Total	6.7	5.0	4.0
	Upright	9.7	6.2	5.0
	Recumbent	2.1	5.3	3.0
Esophageal MII data				
# reflux episodes	Total	73	75	61
	Acid	55	50	51
	Weakly acid	26	33	38
	Weakly alkaline	1	15	18

MII multichannel intraluminal impedance

normal values for an Italian population on a Mediterranean diet [13]. Currently available normal values are summarized in Table 2.2. Using these normal values and the ability to detect non-acid reflux Savarino et al. [21] compared MII-pH findings from 150 patients with typical symptoms and normal upper GI endoscopy (nonerosive reflux disease (NERD)) with those from 48 healthy volunteers. The authors found that NERD patients had more reflux episodes (median [25th–75th percentile]) compared with healthy volunteers (total: 46 [26–65] vs. 32 [18–43], $P<0.05$; acid: 29 [14–43] vs. 17 [8.5–31.0], $P<0.05$; and nonacid: 20 [15–27] vs. 18 [13.5–26.0], P = NS). Among 87 patients with normal distal esophageal acid exposure 22 (15 %) had a positive symptom association probability (SAP) for acid, 19 (12 %) for nonacid reflux, and 7 (5 %) for both. Classifying patients with symptomatic nonacid reflux as having a hypersensitive esophagus reduced the number of patients with functional heartburn from 65 (43 %) to 39 (26 %). These data suggest that monitoring for nonacid reflux in NERD patients reduces the proportion of patients misclassified as having *functional heartburn*.

Early data on post-prandial reflux documented that acid suppressive therapy with PPI reduces distal esophageal acid exposure and number of acid reflux episodes but does not reduce the total number of reflux episodes (Fig. 2.5) [14]. Subsequent studies evaluating acid and non-acid reflux episodes over 24 h noted the same phenomenon that PPI therapy increases the pH of the gastroesophageal refluxate without affecting the total number of reflux episodes. Evaluating 30 patients with typical reflux symptoms on and off PPI therapy Hemmink et al. found fewer acid reflux episodes (49 ± 34 off PPI vs. 20 ± 25 on PPI) but a higher number of weakly acidic reflux episodes (24 ± 17 off PPI vs. 48 ± 31 on PPI) in patients on versus off acid suppressive therapy [15]. By documenting ongoing gastroesophageal reflux in patients on acid suppressive therapy these studies provided a sound rationale for looking for non-acid reflux as a cause of persistent symptoms in the presence of acid suppressive therapy.

Multicenter studies from the US and France documented that in 30–45 % of patients on therapy with PPI twice daily esophageal symptoms during 24-h combined MII-pH monitoring were associated with ongoing gastroesophageal reflux [16, 17]. These studies underscore that non-acid reflux episodes are the main type of reflux associated with persistent symptoms on PPI therapy. In a step-wise increase of acid suppressive therapy in GERD patients Becker et al. [18] evaluated patients with ongoing symptoms while on once daily PPI and found abnormal MII-pH findings (abnormal distal esophageal acid exposure or abnormal number of MII-detected reflux episodes) in 39 % of patients. Patients were followed up for at least 3 months after the dose of PPI was increased. Following increased acid suppression the authors found significantly better symptomatic relief in

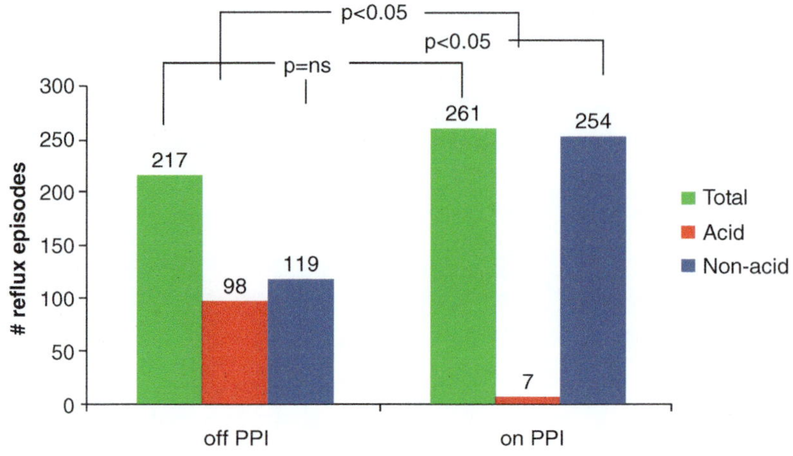

Fig. 2.5 Postprandial gastroesophageal reflux episodes on and off PPI therapy. Acid suppressive therapy reduces the number of acid reflux episodes but does not reduce the total number of reflux episodes. This leads to an apparent paradoxical increase in the number of non-acid (weakly acidic/weakly alkaline) reflux episodes. *PPI* proton pump inhibitor, (Adapted from [14])

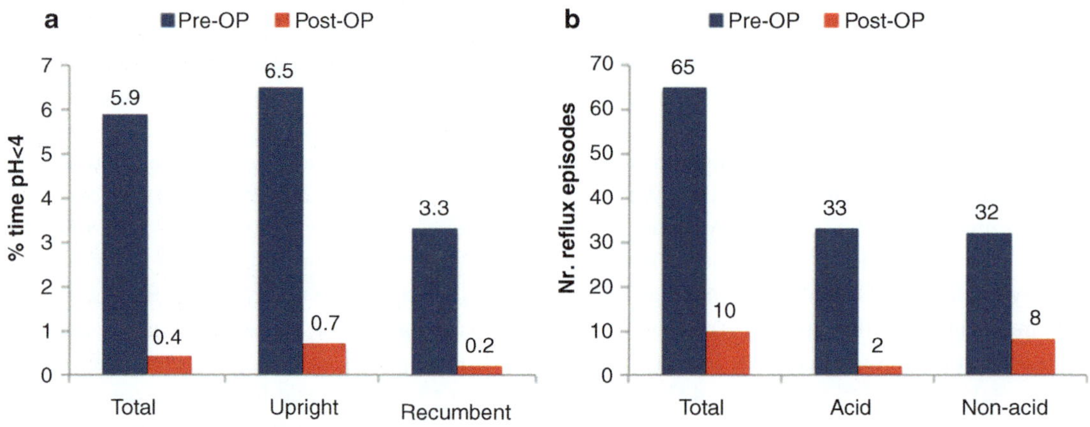

Fig. 2.6 Gastroesophageal reflux before and after Nissen-Rossetti fundoplication. The surgical procedure reduces distal esophageal acid exposure expressed as % time pH<4 (**a**) and all types of gastroesophageal reflux episodes, both acid and non-acid (**b**) (Adapted from [19])

patients with abnormal MII-pH results (90 %) compared to patients with normal MII-pH findings (43 %), concluding that combined MII-pH monitoring facilitates a more focused therapeutic approach to patients with PPI-resistant GERD possibly avoiding PPI overuse.

In contrast to acid suppressive therapy, anti-reflux surgery reduces both acid and non-acid gastroesophageal reflux episodes (Fig. 2.6). Del Genio et al. performed MII-pH monitoring in 15 consecutive patients who underwent laparoscopic Nissen-Rossetti fundoplication before and 7 months after the operation [19]. The authors found not only a significant improvement in esophageal symptoms (heartburn pre-op 2.3 ± 0.8 vs. post-op 0.2 ± 0.2; regurgitation pre-op 1.8 ± 0.9 vs. post-op 0.3 ± 0.2; $p < 0.05$) and distal esophageal acid exposure (total % time pH<4 pre-op 5.9 ± 2.9 vs. post-op 0.4 ± 0.3; $p < 0.05$) but also a significant reduction in the total number of reflux episodes (pre-op 65.2 ± 45.4 vs. post-op 10.0 ± 10.0; $p < 0.01$) both acid (pre-op 33.4 ± 21.4 vs. post-op 1.3 ± 3.6; $p < 0.01$) and non-acid (pre-op 31.8 ± 34.1 vs. post-op 8.3 ± 9.3; $p < 0.05$). Frazzoni et al. documented the superiority of laparoscopic fundoplication over maximal acid suppressive therapy in controlling reflux episodes in patients with persistent symptoms on acid suppressive therapy [20]. Evaluating 71 patients with persistent heartburn/regurgitation on PPI twice daily the authors identified 40 patients with either an increased number of reflux episodes or positive symptom association on acid suppressive therapy prepared to undergo fundoplication. Anti-reflux surgery further reduced distal esophageal acid exposure (% time pH$<$4 on PPI 1.0 (0.3–2.4) vs. post-surgery 0.1 (0.0–0.3); $p<0.01$), and decreased the number of acid (on PPI 14 (6–25) vs. post-surgery 2 (1–6); $p<0.01$) and non-acid reflux episodes (on PPI 69 (50–94) vs. post-surgery 21 (12–31); $p<0.01$).

While these recent data suggest that laparoscopic fundoplication improved gastroesophageal reflux control, other therapeutic options are warranted for patients with persistent symptoms on acid suppressive therapy who are not prepared (or not candidate) for anti-reflux surgery.

2.4 Summary

High resolution esophageal manometry is an important development in esophageal function testing. The increased sensor density and novel topographic representation of pressure changes during swallowing provide a comprehensive evaluation of pharyngeal contraction, upper esophageal sphincter relaxation, esophageal body peristalsis and lower esophageal sphincter relaxation for each swallow. Interpretation of esophageal manometry becomes more intuitive, limiting pitfalls due to LES misplacement, double swallowing or secondary peristalsis. The recent sub-classification of achalasia using HRM makes it possible to predict therapeutic outcome.

Impedance-pH monitoring represents a shift in the reflux monitoring paradigm where reflux episodes are detected as the presence of liquid in the esophagus and sub-classified into acid vs. non-acid (or weakly acidic) based on the pH data. Combined MII-pH monitoring has revealed that non-acid reflux is the main culprit preceding symptoms in patients with persistent symptoms on acid suppressive therapy. This information should allow a better selection of patients who would benefit from therapies aimed at correcting the gastroesophageal barrier such as laparoscopic fundoplication or endoscopic anti-reflux procedures.

Key Points

- Esophageal manometry is indicated in patients with esophageal symptoms and no structural abnormalities (i.e. normal upper GI endoscopy and/or barium esophagogram)
- High resolution manometry provides a detailed description of the upper/lower esophageal sphincter relaxation and esophageal peristalsis during swallowing
- Sub-classification of achalasia allows to predict outcome following pneumatic dilatation or laparoscopic myotomy
- Impedance-pH monitoring detects gastroesophageal reflux episodes independently of their acid content, allowing detection of acid and non-acid reflux
- Non-acid reflux is responsible for ongoing symptoms in up to 40 % of patients under therapy with proton pump inhibitors
- Acid suppressive therapy reduces the acidity of the gastroesophageal refluxate but does not change the total number of gastroesophageal reflux episodes
- Intervention augmenting the gastroesophageal barrier (i.e. laparoscopic fundoplication) is superior to acid suppressive therapy in controlling acid and non acid reflux

References

1. Afkari S (2007) Measuring frequency of spontaneous swallowing. Australas Phys Eng Sci Med 30:313–317
2. Shaheen NJ, Hansen RA, Morgan DR, Gangarosa LM, Ringel Y, Thiny MT, Russo MW, Sandler RS (2006) The burden of gastrointestinal and liver diseases, 2006. Am J Gastroenterol 101:2128–2138
3. Tack J, Fass R (2004) Review article: approaches to endoscopic-negative reflux disease: part of the GERD spectrum or a unique acid-related disorder? Aliment Pharmacol Ther 19(Suppl 1):28–34

4. Spechler SJ, Castell DO (2001) Classification of oesophageal motility abnormalities. Gut 49:145–151
5. Grubel C, Hiscock R, Hebbard G (2008) Value of spatiotemporal representation of manometric data. Clin Gastroenterol Hepatol 6:525–530
6. Ghosh SK, Pandolfino JE, Rice J, Clarke JO, Kwiatek M, Kahrilas PJ (2007) Impaired deglutitive OGJ relaxation in clinical esophageal manometry: a quantitative analysis of 400 patients and 75 controls. Am J Physiol Gastrointest Liver Physiol 293:G878–G885
7. Kahrilas PJ, Ghosh SK, Pandolfino JE (2008) Esophageal motility disorders in terms of pressure topography: the Chicago classification. J Clin Gastroenterol 42:627–635
8. Pandolfino JE, Fox MR, Bredenoord AJ, Kahrilas PJ (2009) Review article: high-resolution manometry in clinical practice: utilizing pressure topography to classify oesophageal motility abnormalities. Neurogastroenterol Motil 21:796–806
9. Bulsiewicz WJ, Kahrilas PJ, Kwiatek MA, Ghosh SK, Meek A, Pandolfino JE (2009) Esophageal pressure topography criteria indicative of incomplete bolus clearance: a study using high-resolution impedance manometry. Am J Gastroenterol 104:2721–2728
10. Pandolfino JE, Kwiatek MA, Nealis TJ, Bulsiewicz W, Post J, Kahrilas PJ (2008) Achalasia: it's not all one disease. Gastroenterology 135:1526–1533
11. Shay SS, Tutuian R, Sifrim D, Vela MF, Wise JL, Balaji NS, Zhang X, Adhami T, Murray JA, Peters JH, Castell DO (2004) Twenty-four hour ambulatory simultaneous impedance and pH monitoring: a multicenter report of normal values from 60 healthy volunteers. Am J Gastroenterol 99:1037–1043
12. Zerbib F, des Varannes SB, Roman S, Pouderoux P, Artigue F, Chaput U, Mion F, Caillol F, Verin E, Bommelaer G, Ducrotté P, Galmiche JP, Sifrim D (2005) Normal values and day-to-day variability of 24-h ambulatory oesophageal impedance-pH monitoring in a Belgian-French cohort of healthy subjects. Aliment Pharmacol Ther 22:1011–1021
13. Zentilin P, Iiritano E, Dulbecco P, Bilardi C, Savarino E, De Conca S, Parodi A, Reglioni S, Vigneri S, Savarino V (2006) Normal values of 24-h ambulatory intraluminal impedance combined with pH-metry in subjects eating a Mediterranean diet. Dig Liver Dis 38:226–232
14. Vela MF, Camacho-Lobato L, Srinivasan R, Tutuian R, Katz PO, Castell DO (2001) Simultaneous intraesophageal impedance and pH measurement of acid and nonacid gastroesophageal reflux: effect of omeprazole. Gastroenterology 120:1599–1606
15. Hemmink GJ, Bredenoord AJ, Weusten BL, Monkelbaan JF, Timmer R, Smout AJ (2008) Esophageal pH-impedance monitoring in patients with therapy-resistant reflux symptoms: ''on' or 'off' proton pump inhibitor? Am J Gastroenterol 103: 2446–2453
16. Mainie I, Tutuian R, Shay S, Vela M, Zhang X, Sifrim D, Castell DO (2006) Acid and non-acid reflux in patients with persistent symptoms despite acid suppressive therapy: a multicentre study using combined ambulatory impedance-pH monitoring. Gut 55:1398–1402
17. Zerbib F, Roman S, Ropert A, des Varannes SB, Pouderoux P, Chaput U, Mion F, Vérin E, Galmiche JP, Sifrim D (2006) Esophageal pH-impedance monitoring and symptom analysis in GERD: a study in patients off and on therapy. Am J Gastroenterol 101:1956–1963
18. Becker V, Bajbouj M, Waller K, Schmid RM, Meining A (2007) Clinical trial: persistent gastro-oesophageal reflux symptoms despite standard therapy with proton pump inhibitors – a follow-up study of intraluminal-impedance guided therapy. Aliment Pharmacol Ther 26:1355–1360
19. del Genio G, Tolone S, del Genio F, Rossetti G, Brusciano L, Pizza F, Fei L, del Genio A (2008) Total fundoplication controls acid and nonacid reflux: evaluation by pre- and postoperative 24-h pH-multichannel intraluminal impedance. Surg Endosc 22:2518–2523
20. Frazzoni M, Conigliaro R, Melotti G (2011) Reflux parameters as modified by laparoscopic fundoplication in 40 patients with heartburn/regurgitation persisting despite PPI therapy: a study using impedance-pH monitoring. Dig Dis Sci 56:1099–1106
21. Savarino E, Zentilin P, Tutuian R, Pohl D, Casa DD, Frazzoni M, Cestari R, Savarino V. The role of nonacid reflux in NERD: lessons learned from impedance-pH monitoring in 150 patients off therapy. Am J Gastroenterol. 2008; 103:2685–93

3 Magnetic Augmentation of the Lower Esophageal Sphincter: Changing the Treatment Paradigm in Patients with Gastroesophageal Reflux Disease

Luigi Bonavina, Greta Saino, Davide Bona,
and Tom R. DeMeester

3.1 Background

Gastroesophageal reflux disease (GERD) is a chronic, progressive condition in which a dysfunction of the lower esophageal sphincter (LES) allows gastric contents to reflux into the esophagus, pharynx, respiratory tract, and mouth. The disease is typically characterized by symptoms of heartburn and regurgitation, and can progress to the complications of erosive esophagitis, Barrett's esophagus and adenocarcinoma. Chronic GERD affects 10 % of the western population and is the leading physician diagnosis in outpatient clinics [1]. The disease creates a correspondingly high burden on the healthcare system and payers, and is cited as a significant contributor to absenteeism and reduced productivity with over $ 9 billion of annual direct costs in the United States alone, the highest cost of any digestive tract disorder [2, 3]. This impact will likely become greater as changes in diet and increasing obesity contribute to a rising incidence of pathological gastroesophageal reflux. The majority of patients with GERD receive adequate relief from proton pump inhibitors (PPIs), but up to 40 % have incomplete relief of symptoms that cannot be addressed by simply increasing the daily dose of medications [4, 5]. Further, it has been shown that patients with a mechanically defective LES are particularly difficult to maintain in a symptom-free state. They have nocturnal acid breakthrough, non-acid reflux, and may progress to complications of the disease, such as position-related regurgitation with aspiration and Barrett's metaplasia, a precursor to adenocarcinoma [6–8].

L. Bonavina (✉) • G. Saino • D. Bona
Department of Biomedical Sciences for Health,
Division of General Surgery,
IRCCS Policlinico San Donato,
University of Milano School of Medicine,
20097 San Donato Milanese (Milan), Italy
e-mail: luigi.bonavina@unimi.it

T.R. DeMeester
Department of Surgery,
Keck School of Medicine,
University of Southern California,
1510 San Pablo St, Suite 514,
Los Angeles, CA 90033, USA

3.2 Rationale for a New Surgical Option

Laparoscopic antireflux surgery has been shown to be a viable alternative to medical treatment in patients with gastroesophageal reflux disease [9]. However, Nissen fundoplication, which is the current surgical gold standard, has a level of technical difficulty and side effects that have limited its use to fewer than 30,000 procedures annually in the United States, corresponding to

L. Bonavina (ed.), *Innovation in Esophageal Surgery*,
DOI 10.1007/978-88-470-2469-4_3, © Springer-Verlag Italia 2012

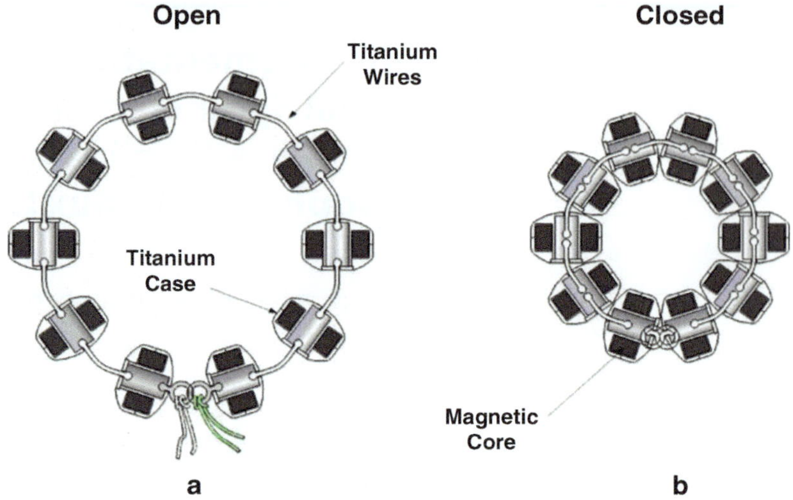

Fig. 3.1 Cross-sectional aspect of the Linx system in open (a) and closed (b) position

less than 1 % of the chronic GERD population [10]. Fundoplication is generally acknowledged to be an effective and durable therapy when performed in specialized centers by surgeons with significant expertise in the treatment of esophageal disease [11–14]; however, outside such centers the success rate varies widely, and reoperative antireflux surgery can be one of the most challenging procedures that a surgeon has to face [15–17]. These factors have contributed to the propensity of patients to persist with pharmacological therapy, even when this has proven inadequate to control symptoms and complications of the disease. Consequently, a significant gap in the treatment continuum for GERD remains evident in the current clinical practice.

3.3 The Concept of Magnetic Sphincter Augmentation

The Linx™ reflux management system is designed to provide a permanent solution to GERD by augmenting the LES barrier with a simple and reproducible laparoscopic procedure that does not alter gastric anatomy and, importantly, can be easily reversed if necessary. The Linx uses magnetic force to augment the natural barrier function of the LES such that for reflux to occur gastric pressures must overcome both the patient's native LES pressure and the magnetic bonds of the device, by this means creating a resistance to sphincter opening. Importantly, the device, while augmenting the LES, also allows for expansion to accommodate a swallowed bolus or the escape of elevated gastric pressure associated with belching or vomiting, thus inhibiting reflux without compromising the physiologic function of the sphincter [18].

The Linx device consists of a series of titanium beads with magnetic cores hermetically sealed inside. This series of beads is interlinked with independent titanium wires to form a flexible ring (Fig. 3.1). The strength of the magnetic core contained in each bead is calibrated by mass to provide a resisting force that precisely augments the sphincter's function. The attractive force between closed beads is approximately 40 g; this decreases exponentially with distance such that the attractive force at full separation is approximately 7 g. At rest, the device encircles the esophago-gastric junction as a "Roman arch", with each magnet resting against its neighbor, to avoid compression of the tubular esophagus. The device is manufactured in different sizes, from 10 to 18 beads, and is capable of nearly doubling its diameter when all beads are separated (Fig. 3.2). Unique to the design is the fact that the magnetic attraction force that must be overcome

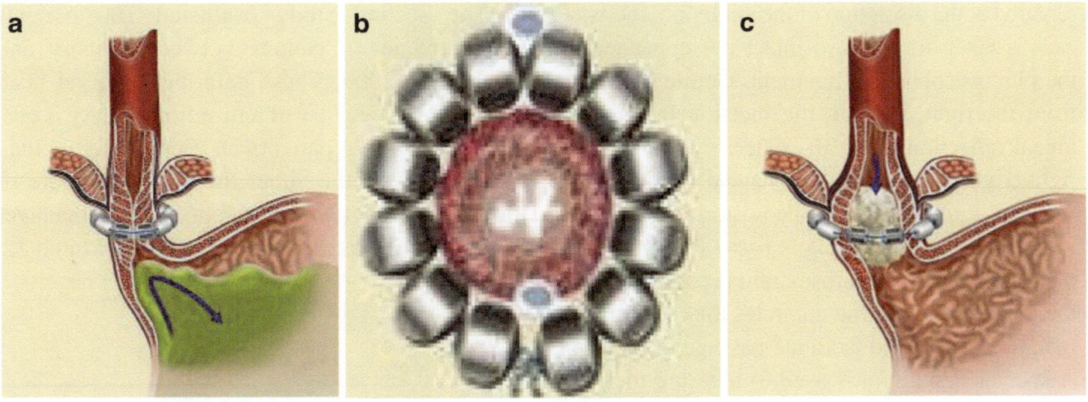

Fig. 3.2 (**a**) The Linx device in closed position; (**b**) the closed position showing no compression of the tubular esophagus; (**c**) the Linx device in open position

Fig. 3.3 Magnetic force response to bead separation

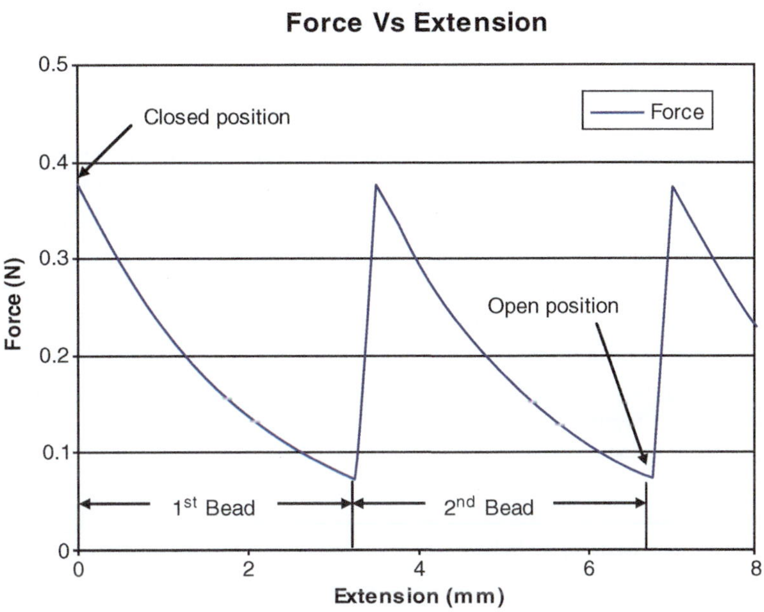

to allow separation of the beads is the same regardless of the number of beads contained in the device (Fig. 3.3).

3.4 Surgical Technique

The Linx device is implanted laparoscopically under general anesthesia. Five ports are typically used for the procedure. With the patient in a 30° reverse Trendelenburg position, the subcardial region is grasped and continuous downward traction is applied. Dissection begins by dividing the peritoneal reflection along the anterior border of the right crus just above the level of the crura decussation. The same dissection is repeated along the left crus. Adipose tissue, if present on the anterior surface of the gastroesophageal junction below the insertion of the inferior leaf of the phrenoesophageal ligament and above the junction of the hepatic branch of the anterior vagus nerve, is divided in a transverse direction to form a trench for the Linx device. If a hernia is present it can be repaired at the discretion of the surgeon; otherwise, care is taken to preserve intact the upper leaf of the phrenoesophageal ligament. Gentle dissection from the right, through the incision in the peritoneal reflection along the anterior border of the right crus, opens a retro-esophageal window and a tunnel is formed between the posterior esophageal wall and the posterior vagus nerve to accomodate the Linx device. A Penrose drain is passed through the posterior tunnel and encircles the esophagus to maintain access and facilitate passage of the Linx. A special sizing tool is used to measure the outer diameter of the esophagus and indicate the size of Linx device to be implanted. Once the appropriate device has been selected, it is introduced through the posterior tunnel. The opposing ends are then brought to the anterior surface of the esophagus, approximated and secured; this completes the implant process.

Operative time is about half an hour. Patients are discharged the day of surgery or on the first post-operative day and instructed to return to a normal diet as tolerated and discontinue the use of acid suppression medications. Patients typically return to normal physical activity in less than a week. The most common complaint following the Linx procedure is mild dysphagia that is easily tolerated and requires only temporary diet adjustments.

3.5 Clinical Trials

Two prospective multi-center and controlled clinical studies have been conducted under a US Food and Drug Administration (FDA) investigational device exemption (IDE G060172) to evaluate the Linx device. The first study evaluated 44 patients implanted at 4 centers with the Linx device between February 2007 and October 2008 [19]. Data from this study were submitted for CE certification and showed the device to have a positive risk-to-benefit ratio. A subsequent publication reported the 2-year results of this study [20]. An additional study evaluating the 4-year results has been recently accepted for publication [21].

The second study evaluated 100 patients implanted at 14 centers between January and September 2009. These data have not yet been published. A registry of anti-reflux surgery is currently enrolling patients in Europe to include treatment with the either the Linx procedure or fundoplication [22]. The Linx reflux management system was approved by FDA on March 22, 2012.

3.6 Published Clinical Experience

The two prospective clinical studies have demonstrated that patients receiving the Linx device have significantly improved quality of life, normalization of reflux, few adverse events and a dramatic reduction in PPI use. As far as concern the feasibility study, the median follow-up time since implantation was 1,343 days (range 119–1,827). Three patients were explanted: one at 226 days post-implant due to persistent dysphagia, the second at 468 days due to the need for a magnetic resonance imaging study, and the third at 1,302 days because of continued GERD symptoms. Surgical removal could be accomplished without difficulty and a Nissen fundoplication was performed in two patients. The mean GERD-health-related quality of life (HRQL) score at 1 year decreased by 85 %, and at 2 years by 90 % ($p < .0001$). At 1 and 2 years 90 and 86 % of the patients were completely off PPI therapy. Mild dysphagia was present in 43 % of patients during the postoperative period, and typically resolved by 90 days without treatment. Esophageal acid exposure was normalized for the total time in 77 and 90 % of patients at 1 and 2 years, respectively. The mean % time pH was <4, decreased from a pre-operative baseline of 11.9–3.1 % at 1 year and 2.4 % at 2 years. All other parameters of the 24-h pH test and the DeMeester composite score were significantly reduced compared to baseline at 1 and 2 years. On upper gastrointestinal endoscopy the impression of the device was observed in the region of the gastroesophageal junction in all patients.

There was no increased resistance to passage of a 9 mm endoscope. No mucosal or transmural erosions of the device were reported. Thirty-two patients had both baseline and 1-year postoperative manometric testing available for comparison. LES resting pressure increased from 6.5 to 14.6 mmHg ($p < .005$) in the nine patients with a hypotensive (less than 10 mmHg) LES pressure. In the 23 patients with normal LES pressure at baseline, no significant changes in pressure occurred. No statistically significant changes in the amplitude of esophageal contractions were observed.

At ≥4-year follow-up, there were no reports of death or long-term related complications. All patients (100 %) had at least a 50 % reduction in the total GERD-HRQL score, and 80 % reported complete cessation of PPI use. Interestingly, a post-hoc questionnaire showed that inability to belch or vomit was reported by less than 5 % (2/44) of the patients.

3.7 Future Perspectives

The limitations of current therapies for GERD have left a significant segment of the reflux patient population in an equivocal position: either to continue with a life-time dependence on a medication that does not provide complete relief of symptoms or have a surgical procedure that requires significant alteration of gastric anatomy, may deteriorate over time and may have significant side effects. Based upon the clinical experience to date, laparoscopic magnetic sphincter augmentation with the Linx device provides patients with a permanent, easily reversible, and more physiologic solution to their reflux. To date, the device has demonstrated a high level of efficacy and has met patient expectations, with few side effects or serious adverse events. If this clinical performance is maintained over the course of the next 5 years, the Linx procedure will become a recognized and significant therapeutic advance in the GERD patient care continuum.

Key Points

- Up to 40 % of patients with gastroesophageal reflux disease report incomplete relief of symptoms despite increasing the daily dose of proton pump inhibitors
- Laparoscopic Nissen fundoplication has traditionally been reserved to patients with advanced disease; further use has been resisted because of the variability in outcomes, the risks of side effects, and the degree of anatomical distortion
- Magnetic sphincter augmentation represents a new standardized surgical option that has been shown to be safe and effective at 4-year follow-up

References

1. Dent J, El-Serag HB, Wallander MA, Johansson S (2005) Epidemiology of gastro-oesophageal reflux disease: a systematic review. Gut 54:710–717
2. Shaheen NJ, Hansen RA, Morgan DR et al (2006) The burden of gastrointestinal and liver diseases, 2006. Am J Gastroenterol 101:2128–2138
3. Thijssen AS, Broeders IA, de Wit GA, Draaisma WA (2011) Cost-effectiveness of proton pump inhibitors versus laparoscopic Nissen fundoplication for patients with gastroesophageal reflux disease: a systematic review of the literature. Surg Endosc 25:3127–3134
4. Dean B, Gano A, Knight K et al (2006) Effectiveness of proton pump inhibitors in nonerosive reflux disease. Clin Gastroenterol Hepatol 2:656–664
5. Sharma N, Agrawal A, Freeman J, Vela M, Castell D (2008) An analysis of persistent symptoms in acid-suppressed patients undergoing impedance-pH monitoring. Clin Gastroenterol Hepatol 6:521–524
6. Lord R, DeMeester S, Peters J, Hagen J, Elyssnia D, Sheth C, DeMeester T (2009) Hiatal hernia, lower esophageal sphincter incompetence, and effectiveness of Nissen fundoplication in the spectrum of gastroesophageal reflux disease. J Gastrointest Surg 13:602–610
7. Vela M, Camacho-Lobato L, Srinivasan R, Tutuian R, Katz P, Castell D (2001) Simultaneous intraesophageal impedance and pH measurement of acid and non-acid gastroesophageal reflux: effect of omeprazole. Gastroenterology 120:1599–1606
8. Peters J, DeMeester T, Crookes P, Oberg S, deVos SM, Hagen J, Bremner C (1998) The treatment of gastroesophageal reflux disease with laparoscopic Nissen

fundoplication. A prospective evaluation of 100 patients with "typical" symptoms. Ann Surg 228:40–50
9. Lundell L (2007) Therapy of gastroesophageal reflux: evidence-based approach to antireflux surgery. Dig Dis 25:188–196
10. Finks JF, Wei Y, Birkmeyer JD (2006) The rise and fall of antireflux surgery in the United States. Surg Endosc 20:1698–1701
11. Dallemagne B, Weerts J, Markiewicz S et al (2006) Clinical results of laparoscopic fundoplication at ten years after surgery. Surg Endosc 20:159–165
12. Kelly JJ, Watson D, Chin KF, Devitt PG, Game PA, Jamieson GG (2007) Laparoscopic Nissen fundoplication: clinical outcomes at 10 years. J Am Coll Surg 205:570–575
13. Oelschlager BK, Quiroga E, Parra JD, Cahill M, Polissar N, Pellegrini C (2007) Long-term outcomes after laparoscopic antireflux surgery. Am J Gastroenterol 102:1–8
14. Morgenthal CB, Shane MD, Stival A et al (2007) The durability of laparoscopic Nissen fundoplication: 11-year outcome. J Gastrointest Surg 11:693–700
15. Vakil N, Shaw M, Kirby R (2003) Clinical effectiveness of laparoscopic fundoplication in a US community. Am J Med 114:1–5
16. Hunter J, Smith C, Branum G et al (1999) Laparoscopic fundoplication failures: patterns of failure and response to fundoplication revision. Ann Surg 230:595–606
17. Smith CD, McClusky DA, Rajad MA et al (2005) When fundoplication fails- redo? Ann Surg 241:861–871
18. Ganz R, Gostout C, Grudem J et al (2008) Use of a magnetic sphincter for the treatment of GERD: a feasibility study. Gastrointest Endosc 67:287–294
19. Bonavina L, Saino G, Bona D et al (2008) Magnetic augmentation of the lower esophageal sphincter: results of a feasibility clinical trial. J Gastrointest Surg 12:2133–2140
20. Bonavina L, DeMeester TR, Fockens P et al (2010) Laparoscopic sphincter augmentation device eliminates reflux symptoms and normalizes esophageal acid exposure. Ann Surg 252:857–862
21. Lipham JC, DeMeester TR, Ganz RA, et al (2012) Apr. 27 PMID: 22538694. The Linx reflux management system: confirmed safety and efficacy now at four years. Surg Endosc
22. Migliore A, Corio M, Paone S, Jefferson T, Cerbo M (2011) Implantable device for patients with gastro-oesophageal reflux disease. Agenas, Agenzia nazionale per i servizi sanitari regionali. Horizon Scanning report no. 9. Agenas, Rome, April 2011. www.agenas.it

4 Transoral Esophageal Myotomy for Achalasia

Karl-Hermann Fuchs, Wolfram Breithaupt, Gábor Varga, and Daniel von Renteln

4.1 Introduction

Patients with achalasia usually present with occasional to persistent dysphagia, regurgitation, retrosternal pain and/or heartburn. The major clinical problem is intermittent obstruction of the esophageal transit of food and/or fluids. The underlying disorder consists of incomplete relaxation of the lower esophageal sphincter during swallowing, increased resting tone of the sphincter, and aperistalsis of the esophageal body.

The therapeutic spectrum of this primary motor disorder consists of medical therapy, endoscopic balloon dilatation, endoscopic Botox-injection, and open or laparoscopic cardiomyotomy. A large meta-analysis found surgical myotomy superior to other treatments regarding the long-term clinical results [1]. A recent randomized trial comparing endoscopic dilatation with laparoscopic myotomy showed similar results after 2 years, when repetitive use of dilation was allowed [2].

More recently, transoral esophageal myotomy has been added to the surgical options. After the idea of creating a submucosal tunnel for endoscopic transmural operations was launched in animal experiments by Pasricha et al. [3], Inoue et al. reported the first experience in humans and introduced per-oral endoscopic myotomy (POEM) into clinical practice [4]. In Europe, von Renteln et al. and Rösch et al. have reported their initial experience with this new technique and confirmed the good early results of Inoue et al. [5].

4.2 Requirements for Establishing POEM in Clinical Practice

The most important requirement is a well experienced team in interventional flexible endoscopy [6]. The endoscopist as well as the assisting staff should have experience in advanced therapeutic endoscopic techniques and hemostasis to handle all necessary endoscopic instruments such as injection needles, needle knife, triangle knife, coagulation graspers and endoscopic clips. During the POEM procedure, there is a certain time pressure, since gas insufflation in the submucosal tunnel is necessary for visualisation,

K.-H. Fuchs (✉) • W. Breithaupt • G. Varga
Department of General-, Visceral- and Thoracic Surgery,
AGAPLESION Markus Krankenhaus,
Frankfurt am Main, Germany
e-mail: karl-hermann.fuchs@fdk.info

D. von Renteln
Department of Endoscopy,
University Hospital Hamburg Eppendorf,
Martinistrasse, Hamburg, Germany

L. Bonavina (ed.), *Innovation in Esophageal Surgery*,
DOI 10.1007/978-88-470-2469-4_4, © Springer-Verlag Italia 2012

which increases the risk of extensive mediastinal, retroperitoneal and subcutaneous emphysema. The prevention of this problem needs quick and safe operative steps with the available flexible endoscopic techniques.

In addition, advanced surgical and especially laparoscopic skills and experience as well as surgical knowledge about esophageal disease must be available in case of conversion and/or consultation. Our team had undergone extensive experimental training in submucosal tunnelling and other natural orifice transluminal endoscopic surgery (NOTES) procedures before introducing this technique into clinical practice.

The necessary equipment consists of the modern endoscopic and laparoscopic technology such as high-resolution video endoscopes and laparoscopes, flexible endoscopic instruments as well as energy sources to provide spray coagulation technique, which is essential for a safe submucosal dissection.

Organisational and legal as well as ethical requirements may vary from country to country and also in different institutions. The evaluation of the protocol to introduce a new innovative technique should be performed by an independent committee such as the institutional review board (IRB), ethical committee or a similar body. It is important to fulfill these requirements when introducing such a potential dangerous procedure, in order to create more safety for all involved: the patient, the endoscopist responsible, the hospital and the method, which has a great potential, if performed safely [7].

4.3 Patient Selection

For the introduction of this new technique, patients with achalasia without prior endoscopic or surgical treatment should be selected in order to ensure optimal tissue conditions in the esophageal wall. The patients should be able to understand the procedure well and should also be able to understand the possible risk of complications with such a new technique as well as the advantages and disadvantages. The investigators who initially published their experience emphasized the importance of informing the patient adequately. In Europe, the requirements in the different countries may vary remarkably regarding informed consent and IRB approval.

4.4 Technique of POEM

Prior to the operation the patient must have fasted for 8 h. During the 3 days before the procedure the patient is instructed to eat only semisolid food and drink sufficiently to prevent food obstruction in the esophagus above the cardia.

The procedure is performed under general anesthesia. The patient is placed in the supine position and the abdomen is free for inspection and palpation during the procedure to check the possible presence of a pneumoperitoneum. In this case, a Veress needle is inserted under sterile conditions to release the carbon dioxide (CO_2) gas from the abdominal cavity. The infection-contamination issue is addressed by discontinuing all antisecretory drugs 1 week prior to the operation in order to keep the intragastric environment as acidic as possible and reduce bacterial growth. Antibiotic prophylaxis (ciprofloxacin and metronidazole) is given intravenously. After the operation, high dose proton pump inhibitors are routinely administered.

Prior to the actual procedure, the upper gastrointestinal tract is checked with an endoscope to remove all fluid and/or residual food from the esophageal lumen. The esophageal, pharyngeal and gastric lumen is extensively rinsed with chlorhexidine.

The patient is covered with sterile drapes up to the mouth. Then a gastroscope is introduced into the esophagus attached to a CO_2 insufflator. A transparent cap is attached to the tip of the scope for better exposure. Initially the important esophageal landmarks are measured, e.g. the distal end of the cardia, and the narrowing of the cardia in the distal esophagus, representing

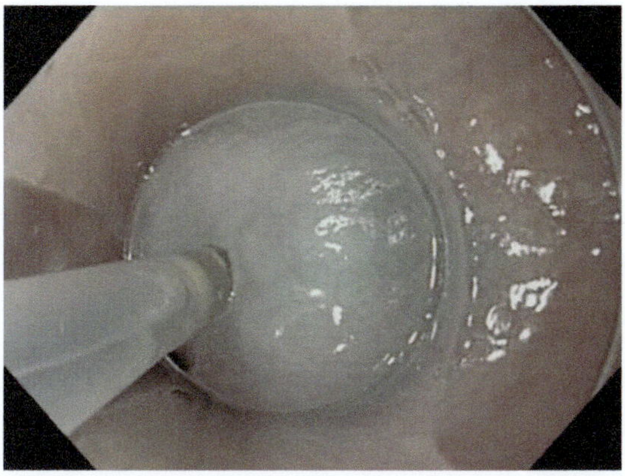

Fig. 4.1 Submucosal injection and lifting of the esophageal mucosa 5 cm above the planned starting point of the myotomy

the upper end of the non-relaxing high-pressure zone. The myotomy should start a few centimeters above the latter area. Thus, the mucosal entry will be about 5 cm above the starting point of the myotomy, if one aims for a safe tunnel distance of 5 cm. Usually this entry myotomy site is located between 28 and 32 cm from the teeth.

After the measurements, 5–10 ml of blue-stained saline and epinephrine will be injected into the submucosal area (Fig. 4.1). This will lift the mucosa from the muscular layer and facilitate the mucosal incision with a triangle-tip knife that creates the entrance into the tunnel (Fig. 4.2). Further alternating injection of blue-stained saline, application of spray-coagulation, and moderate pushing of the endoscope will complete the tunnel down to the area below the cardia (Fig. 4.3). These steps should be performed with extreme care and caution in order to prevent damage to the mucosa, which is the only intact layer protecting the mediastinum once the myotomy is completed.

It is important to remove the endoscope from the tunnel several times to double-check the correct direction of the tunnel within the esophageal circumference as well as the advancement of the tunnel towards and below the cardia. A final check should include an endoscopic retroflex view to confirm the blue-stained gastric mucosa at the end of the tunnel below the cardia.

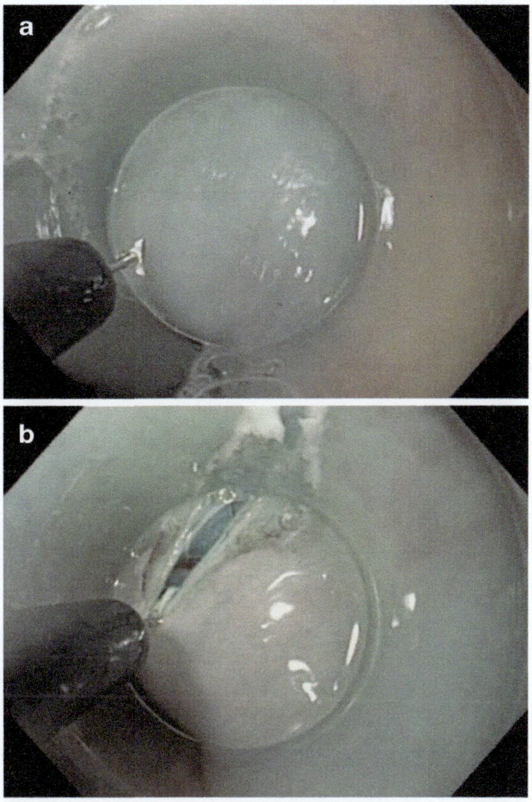

Fig. 4.2 Creation of the mucosal entry site

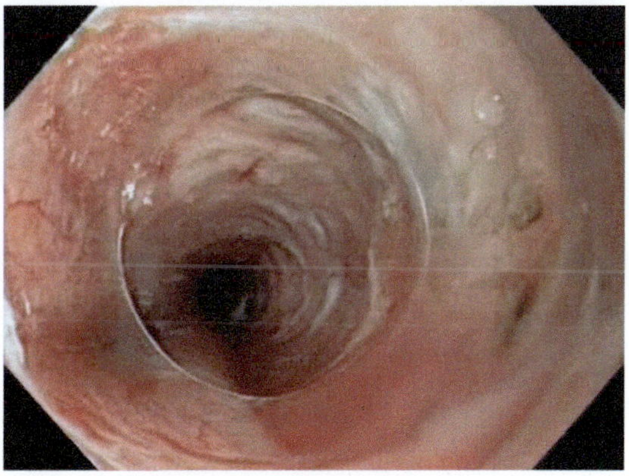

Fig. 4.3 Development of the submucosal tunnel

Then the endoscope is repositioned in the tunnel at the starting point of the myotomy and the myotomy is advanced distally with the triangle-tip knife, possibly severing only the circular layer of the muscle and leaving the longitudinal muscle

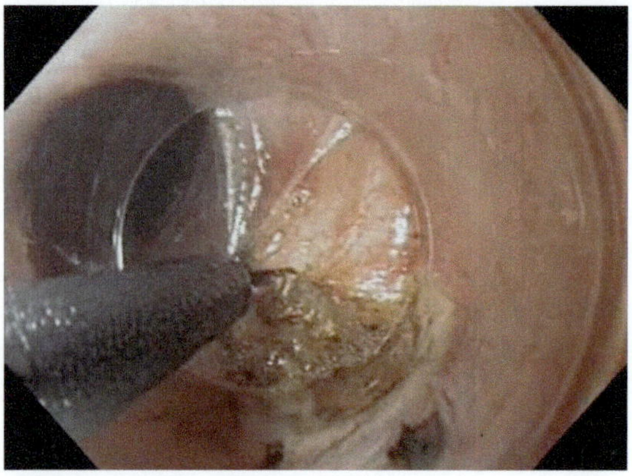

Fig. 4.4 Endoscopic submucosal myotomy

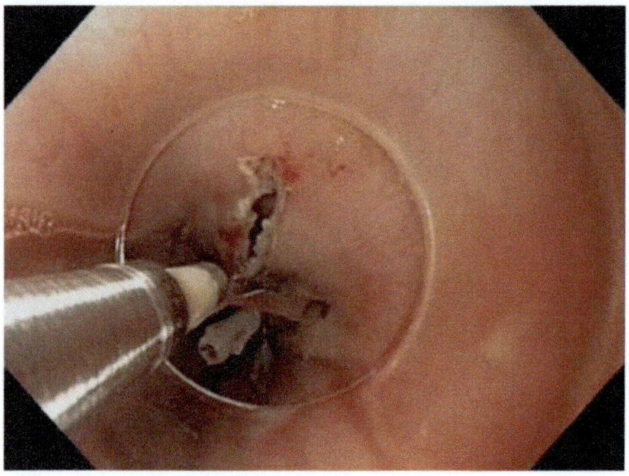

Fig. 4.5 Closure of the mucosal entry site with multiple clips

fibers intact (Fig. 4.4). At the end of the procedure, the extent of the myotomy is checked, all fluids are sucked out of the tunnel and the mucosal defect is closed by clips (Fig. 4.5).

Conclusions

In Europe, only a few centers with large experience in esophageal disease, laparoscopy and advanced interventional endoscopy have introduced this POEM technique in clinical practice. The initial success and the low complication rates are quite promising and show great future prospects for this technique.

Key Points

- Laparoscopic Heller myotomy plus anterior fundoplication is the standard surgical therapy for achalasia with well established long-term results
- Per-oral endoscopic myotomy has recently been introduced and developed in a few specialized centers
- Selective incision of the circular muscle fibers and keeping intact the phrenoesophageal ligament are expected to reduce the incidence of postoperative gastroesophageal reflux

References

1. Campos GM, Vittinghoff E, Rabel C et al (2009) Endoscopic and surgical treatments of achalasia: a system review and meta-analysis. Ann Surg 249:45–57
2. Boeckxstaens GE, Annese V, des Varannes SB et al (2011) Pneumatic dilatation versus laparoscopic Heller's myotomy for idiopathic achalasia. N Engl J Med 364:1807–1816
3. Pasricha PJ, Hawari R, Ahmed I et al (2007) Submucosal endoscopic esophageal myotomy: a novel experimental approach for the treatment of achalasia. Endoscopy 39:761–764
4. Inoue H, Minami H, Kobayashi Y et al (2010) Peroral endoscopic myotomy (POEM) for esophageal achalasia. Endoscopy 42:265–271
5. von Renteln D, Inoue H, Minami H, Werner YB, Pace A, Kersten JF, Much CC, Schachschal G, Mann O, Keller J, Fuchs KH, Rösch T (2012) Peroral endoscopic myotomy for the treatment of achalasia: a prospective single center study. Am J Gastroenterol 107:411–417
6. Rattner DM, Hawes R, Schwaitzberg S, Kochmann M, Swanstrom L (2011) The second SAGES/ASGE white paper on natural orifice transluminal endoscopic surgery: 5 years of progress. Surg Endosc 25:2441–2448
7. Neugebauer EA, Becker M, Buess GF, Cuschieri A, Dauben HP, Fingerhut A, Fuchs KH, Habermalz B, Lantsberg L, Morino M, Reiter-Theil S, Soskuty G, Wayand W, Welsch T (2010) EAES recommendations on methodology of innovation management in endoscopic surgery. Surg Endosc 24:1594–1615

5 Radiofrequency Ablation and Antireflux Management for Non-dysplastic Barrett's Esophagus

Stephanie Fischer See, Sebastian F. Schoppmann, Martin Riegler, and Johannes Zacherl

5.1 Introduction

Barrett's esophagus (BE), i.e. columnar lined esophagus with intestinal metaplasia, develops as a consequence of gastroesophageal reflux disease (GERD) [1]. The diagnosis requires endoscopy and biopsy sampling of the esophagogastric junction. During endoscopy, the esophagogastric junction is considered normal if the squamocolumnar junction coincides with the level of the rise of the gastric type (rugal) folds [2, 3]. The presence of endoscopically visible segments, tongues and islands of columnar type mucosa within the tubular esophagus defines endoscopically visible columnar lined esophagus (CLEv) [4, 5]. If biopsies from CLEv contain intestinal metaplasia (i.e. goblet cells) the condition is termed Barrett's esophagus without dysplasia [2, 3] (Fig. 5.1). Depending on the length of the CLEv-segment, Barrett's esophagus has been defined as long- (>3 cm) or short-segment (≤3 cm) [2, 3]. Presence of intestinal metaplasia within biopsies obtained from an endoscopically normal appearing esophagogastric junction defines ultra-short Barrett's esophagus (i.e. CLE not visible to the resolution of the endoscope) [1, 2]. In GERD patients the likelihood of non-dysplastic Barrett's esophagus (NDBE) increases with increasing length of CLEv and approximates 25, 50 and 100 % for normal junction, CLEv ≤ 3.0 and > 5.0 cm, respectively [3].

Columnar lined esophagus (CLE) results from gastroesophageal reflux. Medical therapy alters the pH of the reflux [6], but does not affect the occurrence of reflux *per se* [7]. Thus the esophagus remains exposed to a more alkaline reflux, which is suggested to propagate the tissue stress and the development of dysplasia and cancer [8, 9]. In contrast to the medical therapy, effective surgery creates an anti-reflux mechanism, which impairs both acid and non acid reflux [10, 11]. In theory, elimination of the reflux should foster cancer prevention.

Via a multi-step sequence involving low- (LGD) and high grade dysplasia (HGD), non-dysplastic Barrett's esophagus (NDBE) may progress to esophageal adenocarcinoma (0.5 % annual risk, i.e. 1 in 10 people with NDBE will develop esophageal cancer within 20 years) [1, 5, 12]. Endoscopic screening and surveillance aim to detect individuals with NDBE and to treat premalignant stages of the disease [13]. Current cancer prevention concentrates on *symptomatic* NDBE and the corresponding elimination of

S.F. See
Manometry Lab, University Clinic of Surgery, Medical University Vienna, Vienna, Austria

S.F. Schoppmann • J. Zacherl
Department of General Surgery, University Clinic of Surgery, Medical University Vienna, Vienna, Austria

M. Riegler (✉)
University Clinic of Surgery, Medical University Vienna, Vienna General Hospital, Vienna, Austria
e-mail: franz.riegler@meduniwien.ac.at

L. Bonavina (ed.), *Innovation in Esophageal Surgery*,
DOI 10.1007/978-88-470-2469-4_5, © Springer-Verlag Italia 2012

dysplasia/early cancer [13]. However, the pathogenesis of CLE justifies to consider *active* treatment at the stage of non-dysplastic Barrett's esophagus and an effective anti-reflux surgery for the elimination of all gastroesophageal reflux [1, 3, 14]. Finally, the epidemiology of esophageal adenocarcinoma suggests that screening should be extended to individuals without GERD symptoms [15]. At this point let us focus some light on the genesis of columnar lined esophagus and see how these insights translate into clinical management.

5.2 Neurohumoral Orchestration of Columnar Lined Esophagus

Following a holistic approach, gastroesophageal reflux activates a complex neurohumoral response within the esophageal mucosa, involving epithelial-, nerve-, vascular-, immune-cells, myofibroblasts, and mediators released from these cells (neuropeptides, growth factors, interleukins), which orchestrates the development of CLE [16] (Fig. 5.2). The reflux-induced neurohumoral flush causes inflammation and replacement of the normal squamous epithelium by a columnar lining consisting of mucus cells only, termed *cardiac mucosa* (CM) [17, 18]. By inclusion of parietal cells, CM may turn into oxyntocardiac mucosa (OCM), or, by inclusion of goblet cells, into non-dysplastic Barrett's esophagus (NDBE) [17, 18]. While OCM harbors no cancer risk [5], the presence of goblet cells within cardiac mucosa indicates the possibility for progression towards NDBE (i.e. cardiac mucosa constitutes a precursor of NDBE) [5, 17]. The histopathological changes are preceded by genetic alterations within the mucosa, which format the epithelium for CLE and cancer development [1, 19, 20]. The endoscopically normal-appearing squamous lined esophagus of Barrett's patients expresses the genetic markers required for the development of NDBE (CDx2, BMP-4) [19, 20]. In a similar manner, the genetic changes required for the development of dysplasia and cancer are already expressed within NDBE (aneuploidy; CDx2;

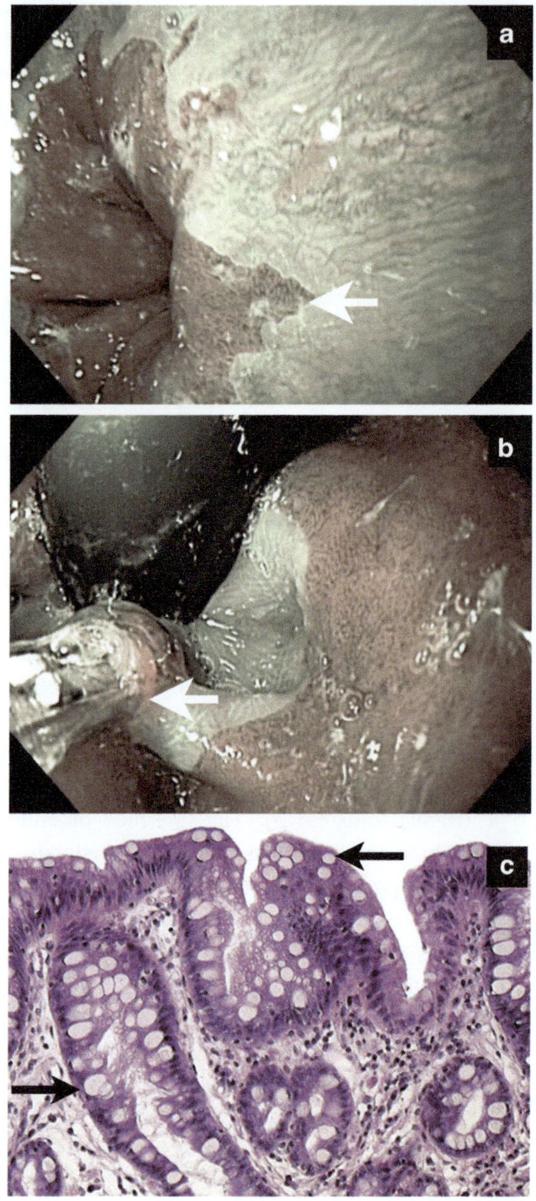

Fig. 5.1 Narrow band imaging endoscopy (**a**, **b**) and histopathology (**c**) of non-dysplastic Barrett's esophagus. (**a**) Antegrade view towards an irregular squamocolumnar junction (*white arrow*). (**b**) Retroflexed view towards the squamocolumnar junction during biopsy sampling. The biopsy forceps straddles the squamocolumnar junction (*white arrow*). (**c**) Histopathology obtained from the irregular squamocolumnar junction shows columnar epithelium containing goblet cells (*black arrows*), the hallmark of non-dysplastic Barrett's esophagus (H&E stain, Courtesy of Prof. Dr. F. Wrba and Dr. I. Mesteri, Vienna). (**a**, **b**) Endoscopy using narrow band imaging (*NBI*) technology, Olympus, Austria

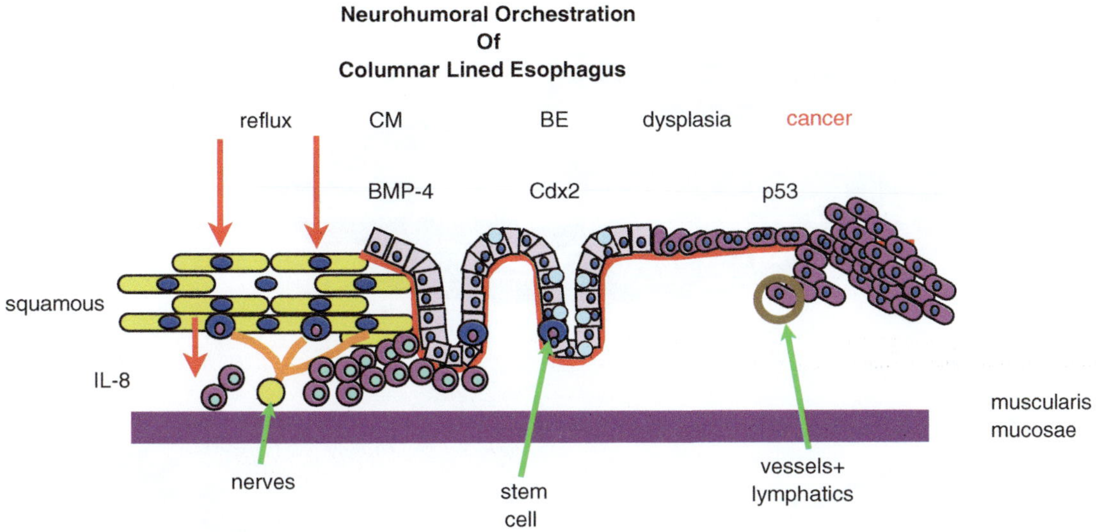

Fig. 5.2 The image cartoons the development of columnar lined esophagus, as described in the text. The reflux-induced neurohumoral flush formats the genetic changes towards non-dysplastic Barrett's esophagus, dysplasia and cancer. BMP-4 drives the formation of columnar epithelium, CDx2 mediates the formation of goblet cells containing intestinal mucosa (i.e. Barrett's esophagus without dysplasia). P53 drives the progression towards dysplasia and cancer. *IL-8*, interleukin 8. Stem cells give rise to columnar cell line (Ref. [12, 16])

p16-, p53-abnormalities and EGFR abnormalities) [1, 12, 19, 20]. Thus, NDBE definitely harbors the genetic information for dysplasia and cancer [12]. However, nobody knows when and where within a given segment of CLE this information will express at the protein level and give rise to the development of the dysplastic epithelium [12]. The complex interaction between reflux and the CLE-orchestra triggers the genetic and morphologic responses leading to the development of dysplasia and cancer [12, 16]. Consequently the possibility remains that this oncologic mucosal "powder keg" could explode.

In line with the pathogenesis of GERD and NDBE, the therapy aims to eradicate the tissue at risk for cancer development and to eliminate the cause of the disease, i.e. gastroesophageal captured. Conceptually these issues should be well catered for by radiofrequency ablation (RFA) [21] and anti reflux surgery [10], for the removal of the premalignant CLE and the elimination of the reflux [14], respectively. Medical therapy is highly effective in a significant number of patients to eliminate GERD symptoms [6], but instead of eliminating the reflux, proton pump inhibitor (PPI) therapy works by altering the pH of the reflux, as assessed by impedance-pH monitoring (reflux monitoring) [7]. Here we briefly describe the principles of RFA and antireflux surgery and their impact on the control of symptomatic NDBE.

5.3 Radiofrequency Ablation: What It Is and How It Works

Radiofrequency ablation (RFA)(HALO®, BarrX, CA, USA) represents a novel endoscopic technique for durable elimination of columnar lined esophagus (CLE) containing non-dysplastic Barrett's esophagus (NDBE), dysplasia and early cancer [12, 21] (Fig. 5.3). Short pulses of radiofrequency energy are applied to "burn" the abnormal esophageal mucosa, without affecting deeper layers of the esophagus (submucosa). Thus the integrity and function of the esophagus are retained. The ablated areas are resealed by a histopathologically and genetically normal mucosa in more than 70 and 95 % of the cases after the 1st and 2nd–4th treatment, respectively. Since RFA includes the entire mucosa it eliminates the target cells for

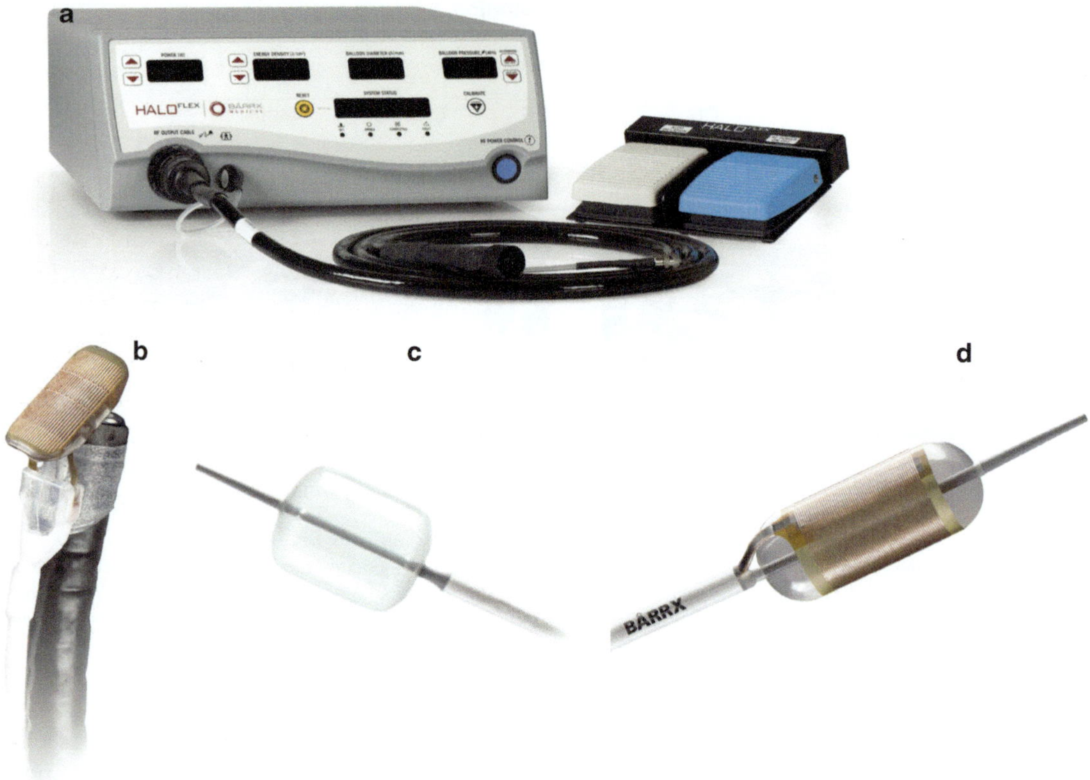

Fig. 5.3 Equipment for radiofrequency ablation (*RFA*) of Barrett's esophagus includes the HALOflex generator (**a**), foot pedal (**a**), HALO^{90} device for focal ablation (**b**), sizing balloon (**c**), HALO^{360} treatment balloon for circumferential ablation (**d**) (Images provided with permission of BarrX Medical, CA, USA)

cancer development (the epithelial cells) and the compartment generating the *neurohumoral flush* (the *lamina propria mucosae*) [16, 21].

The radiofrequency energy (RF energy) is delivered to the mucosa via a balloon catheter based system for the circumferential ablation (HALO$^{360®}$) (Figs. 5.3 and 5.4) and an endoscope tip-mounted plate for focal ablation of endoscopically visible tongues, segments and islands of columnar mucosa within the esophagus (HALO$^{90®}$). Both procedures can be conducted under deep sedation or general anesthesia. We recommend an overnight stay after the ablation for the medical therapy of rare post-interventional side effects (pain, fever, vomiting, nausea). Post-RFA swallow x-ray is recommended for the exclusion of perforation and stenosis. Perforation is rare and may be managed by either stent placement without or with concomitant laparoscopic fundoplication [21].

The RFA technology consists of (Fig. 5.3):

- the foot pedal operated generator (HALOflex®; delivers the RF energy);
- guidewire for introduction of the balloon catheter;
- the HALO^{360} balloon (18, 22, 25, 28, 31 mm diameter); balloon length 4 cm; electrode length 3 cm;
- the HALO sizing balloon (to assess diameter of the treatment balloon), balloon length 4 cm;
- the HALO^{90}: 20.62 mm length, 13.21 mm width; active electrode dimensions: 20 mm length, 13 mm width; recommended scope dimensions: 8.6–12.8 mm;
- HALO-procedure record sheet® to protocol the endoscopic landmarks, procedural steps

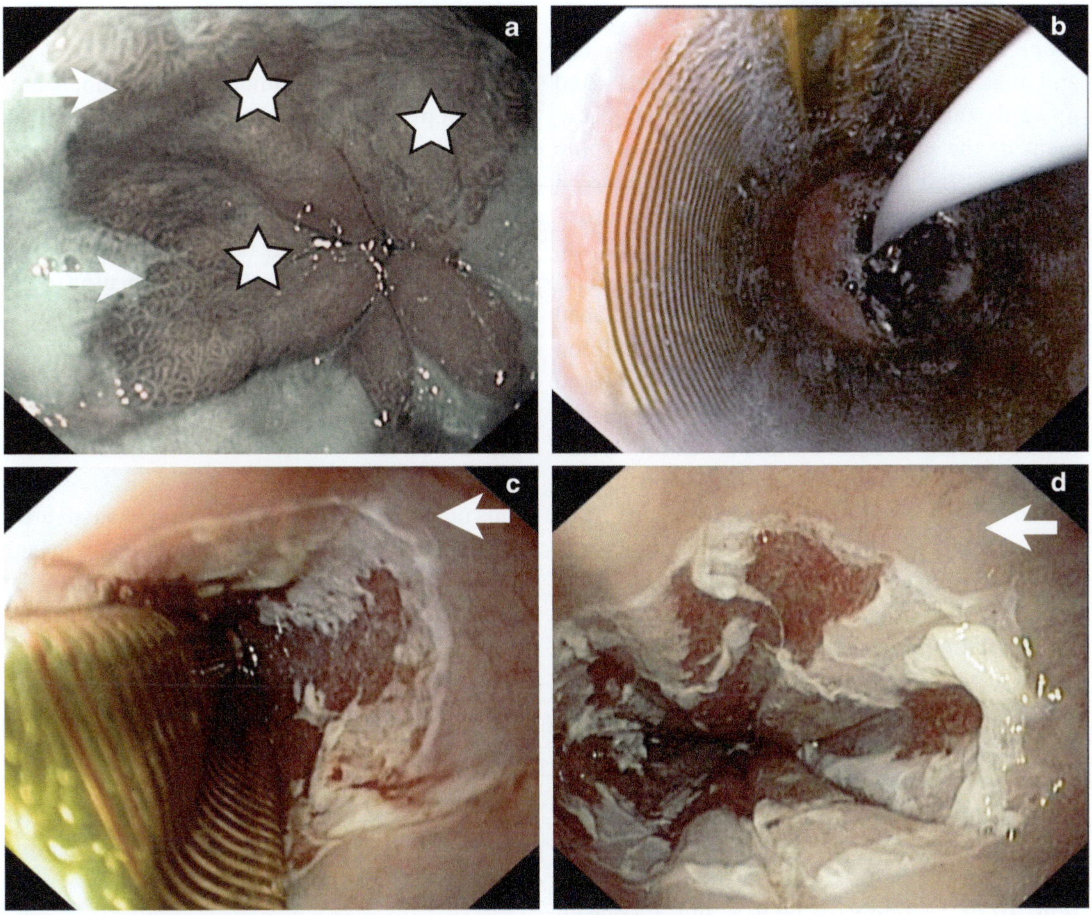

Fig. 5.4 Antegrade endoscopic images of the distal esophagus before (**a**), during (**b**) and after radiofrequency ablation (**c**, **d**) of non-dysplastic Barrett's esophagus. (**a**) Endoscopically visible irregular squamocolumnar junction (*white arrows*) adjacent to the level of the rise of the gastric type folds (*asterisks*). (**b**) Endoscopic vision through the inflated HALO^{360} balloon during the administration of the first pulse of radiofrequency energy to the mucosa. (**c**) Following desufflation the treatment balloon collapses and gives vision to the ablated segment of esophageal mucosa (*white arrow* marks the proximal limit of the ablated area). (**d**) endoscopic image of the distal esophagus after the administration of the second pulse of radiofrequency energy (*white arrow* marks the proximal limit of the ablated area). (**a**) Endoscopy using narrow band imaging (*NBI*) technology, Olympus, Austria. (**b**, **c**) HALO^{360} balloon catheter (BarrX Medical, CA, USA)

(check list), sizing balloon data, diameter of the treatment balloon and/or use of the electrode for the focal ablation.

5.3.1 HALO^{360} Procedure

All procedural steps and data (endoscopic landmarks, esophageal diameter, size of the treatment balloon) assessed during the procedure are catalogued on the HALO-procedure record sheet. Following endoscopic assessment of the level of the squamocolumnar junction (SCJ) and the level of the rise of the endoscopically visible gastric type folds (given as cm from the incisors) (Fig. 5.4a), acetylcystein is applied to the lumen of the distal esophagus for the removal of the mucous layer, which impedes the distribution of RF energy within the tissue. The level of the rise of the gastric type folds is recorded and the endoscope is moved forward into the duodenum for the placement of the guidewire via the working channel of the endoscope. Be sure that the guidewire stays in place and that its tip does not dislocate and wind upwards into the esophagus. Incorrect placement of the guidewire may foster fosse route formation and perforation. Following removal of the endoscope, the sizing balloon is introduced via the guidewire and placed 12 cm above the rise of the gastric type folds (e.g. if the folds rise 40 cm, the sizing balloon is placed at 28 cm from the incisors). The sizing balloon is connected to the generator, calibrated and the diameter of the distal 12 cm of the esophagus is assessed in 1.0 cm increments via foot-pedal activation. The diameter of the esophagus as actually measured and the recommended balloon size are depicted on the display of the HALOflex generator and catalogued on the HALO record sheet. Following removal of the sizing balloon, the treatment balloon with the smallest recommended diameter is inserted via the guidewire into the esophagus. Under endoscopic vision the treatment balloon is placed with its proximal limit at the level of the squamocolumnar junction, inflated (by foot pedal activation) and the RF energy pulse is delivered to the mucosa (by foot pedal activation, 10 or 12 J/cm^2 for NDBE and dysplasia, respectively; the energy pulse is automatically terminated by the generator) (Fig. 5.4b). Thus ablation is conducted in 3 cm steps until the distal level of the CLE is reached, i.e. the level of the rise of the gastric type folds (max. 9 cm per session recommended). In the case of a normal endoscopic junction a single 3 cm long segment is ablated.

After the first ablation circle the necrotic mucosa is scraped off from the mucosal surface, using an endoscope tip mounted plastic cap. Then the second ablation circle is conducted to eliminate remnant CLE glands. Cleaning of the esophageal luminal surface is essential to improve the effect of the second treatment circle. A brown-red color of the luminal surface of the esophagus indicates an effective treatment depth with removal of the entire mucosa. Necrotic tissue adheres to the esophageal wall (Fig. 5.4d). Following deflation of air from the stomach and esophagus, the HALO^{60} treatment balloon is withdrawn under endoscopic vision. The entire procedure lasts approximately 20–30 min. A final endoscopy documents the treated area, excludes submucosal laceration or bleeding, and makes sure that the air is removed from the stomach and esophagus. The proximal and distal limit of the treated segment should be documented (on the HALO protocol sheet). The information helps to target the biopsy levels during the follow up endoscopy (see below).

5.3.2 HALO^{90}

This device is used for the ablation of small areas of endoscopically visible CLE containing intestinal metaplasia (either for first treatment or for the removal of recurrent NDBE after HALO^{360} ablation). The HALO^{90} electrode is connected to the generator, mounted on the tip of the endoscope and thus moved forward to the treatment area. For each area two pulses of 12/cm^2 are applied to the mucosa, followed by removal of the necrotic mucosa and administration of two additional RF energy pulses. Indications and contraindications for RFA are listed in Tables 5.1 and 5.2.

Table 5.1 Preconditions for radiofrequency ablation of symptomatic non-dysplastic Barrett's esophagus (NDBE)

Evidence of NDBE in esophageal biopsies
Positive family history for upper gastrointestinal tract (esophagus, stomach), colorectal, hepato-biliopancreatic cancer
Age < 50 years and absence of comorbidities
Long standing GERD (>5 years)
Absence of contraindications

Table 5.2 Contraindications of radiofrequency ablation

Structural abnormalities of the esophagus (ulcer, stenosis, stricture, diverticula, webs, rings, tumor, polyps, severe inflammation)
Pregnancy
Comorbidities (heart, lungs, rheuma, connective tissue disease, other malignancies)
Anti blood clotting medications
Cardiac pace maker
Mental illness, inability to sign written consent

5.4 Follow up Endoscopy and Biopsy Sampling

Following RFA treatment the patients are put on high dose PPI therapy (i.e. 2×40 mg p.o. daily) for 1 year, then symptom based PPI treatment is continued. Eight to 10 weeks after RFA, endoscopy assesses the effect of ablation; in the case of relapse of Barrett's esophagus (endoscopy- and histopathology-proven) additional HALO^{360} or HALO^{90} treatment(s) is (are) performed until the successful elimination of Barrett's esophagus. Following RFA treatment after effective fundoplication, PPI therapy is administered for 4 weeks and then discontinued.

Annual follow up endoscopies are recommended after effective elimination of non-dysplastic Barrett's esophagus (NDBE) [12, 21].

According to the treatment protocol, the post RFA biopsies should include the entire length of the treated segment in 1.0 cm increments, irrespective of the endoscopic appearance, to exclude the presence of disease recurrence (NDBE) and the formation of buried glands underneath normal squamous lining of the esophagus.

5.5 Effectiveness of Radiofrequency Ablation for the Elimination of Non-dysplastic Barrett's Esophagus

Elimination of Barrett's esophagus is defined as the absence of endoscopically visible and histopathological NDBE after RFA. Going in line with the observations made after treatment of dysplasia and early cancer (>80 % elimination after 2 years; mean 3–4 RFA sessions required, cancers prevented) [22, 23], RFA was highly effective in eliminating non-dysplastic Barrett's esophagus [24–26]. In addition, those studies showed that the neo-squamous epithelium lacks genetic abnormalities [27] and that RFA did not impair esophageal function, as assessed by esophageal manometry [28].

Fleischer et al. [24] demonstrated that elimination of NDBE was achieved in 70 % of the cases after the first treatment session; the other patients required two to four more RFA treatments for complete eradication of NDBE. This effect was durable as 92 % of patients were free of NDBE 5 years after RFA [26]. The residual 8 % with relapse of NDBE underwent an additional RFA therapy. Thus in all patients NDBE was eliminated, and none progressed to dysplasia or cancer [26]. Comparable data were found in other multi-center studies, confirming the efficacy of RFA for the elimination of NDBE [25]. Finally, RFA for NDBE has also been demonstrated to be cost effective [29]. A recent analysis indicated that 45 cases of NDBE are to be treated to prevent one esophageal adenocarcinoma in the subsequent 5 years (13 cases of low grade dysplasia are to be treated to prevent 1 cancer) [12].

After RFA adequate biopsy sampling includes the endoscopically normal-appearing squamous epithelium adjacent to the neo-squamo-columnar junction to exclude the formation of so-called buried CLE glands underneath the squamous epithelium. A recent meta-analysis found that so-called buried glands were reported in 0.9 % of the cases after RFA [30].

Taken together, RFA reverts genetic and morphological abnormalities of NDBE, dysplasia and early cancer [27]. The question remains how this translates into cancer prevention, and where in the sequence from NDBE to cancer RFA should be implemented in order to prevent cancer development.

5.6 Morbidity and Side-Effects of RFA

Complications following RFA for the management of NDBE are rare and include perforation, stricture formation, bleeding, nausea, vomiting, bradycardia, heartburn and chest pain (0.01–1.2 % of cases) [12, 22–26]. Strictures adequately respond to balloon dilatation; the other side effects are successfully managed by medical therapy [22–26]. The frequency of stricture formation after RFA increases with advanced disease: 6.0 % stricture formation and 4.0 % severe complications (hemorrhage, severe chest pain, severe nausea) in patients who underwent RFA for the elimination of dysplasia [22, 23].

5.7 Why Ablate Non-dysplastic Barrett's Esophagus?

Esophageal adenocarcinoma develops along a multi-step sequence via multilayered epithelium, cardiac mucosa, NDBE, low- and high-grade dysplasia [1, 12]. Conceptually, cancer could be prevented by stopping the process at any stage prior to the development of cancer. However, NDBE is associated with fundamental diagnostic and prognostic uncertainties, which are mainly due to the biological, genetic and morphological characteristics of Barrett's esophagus [12].

For an individual the duration of the presence of NDBE is unknown, as well as the duration until progression to cancer. NDBE is not a uniform lesion [2, 5, 17, 18]. Although Barrett's esophagus starts at the squamocolumnar junction the different epithelial types form in a mosaic-like manner [5, 17, 18]. Thus, up to 50 % of the cases with high-grade dysplasia harbor a heterotopic cancer within their CLE [17, 18]. This reflects the potential underscoring of the disease due to biopsy sampling error, and advanced stages (dysplasia, cancer) of the disease may be missed [12]. Next, inter-observer variability contributes to up or down grading of a lesion. When compared to the general population (3 per 100,000) [31], persons with NDBE, low- and high-grade dysplasia harbor a 200×, 560× and 2,200× increased risk for cancer development.

The genetic and molecular abnormalities assessed in NDBE are similar to those found in dysplasia and cancer (p53, p16, CDx2, aneuploidy, lack of apoptosis) [12]. It is not known when these changes will express at the protein level to give rise to the formation of dysplasia and cancer. Most importantly, genetic abnormalities characteristic of dysplasia have been found within CLE without goblet cells [12]. In addition it has been suggested that the stage of NDBE can be bypassed during cancer formation, i.e. that the stage of goblet cells containing CLE is not required for cancer formation [32]. These uncertainties impair the life quality and productivity of the patients (fear to get cancer) and contribute to the diagnostic and therapeutic dilemma of the physician.

Effective and durable removal of NDBE will eliminate the above problems. Without NDBE there is no need to think about cancer risk, biopsy sampling error, inter observer variability, or genetic and DNA abnormalities. However, we have to ensure that the patient undergoes regular follow up endoscopies, to exclude neo-NDBE formation. If this does happen, elimination of the NDBE will keep us on the safe side.

The alternative to this approach is to "wait and see" until dysplasia and early cancer develop. At this stage it becomes difficult for the physician (complex interventions) and dangerous for the patient (increased diagnostic insecurity, procedure-induced complications, inability to reverse the genetic and DNA abnormalities). Accordingly, the wait and see policy did not impair the increase of the frequency of esophageal adenocarcinoma [7]. Finally, the risk of NDBE to progress to cancer is comparable to the cancer risk of a colorectal polyp [12, 13]. Thus NDBE should be offered a strategy comparable to that of the colorectal polyps: act and remove.

Taken together, esophageal adenocarcinoma is the only cancer where the precursor lesions are well-characterized, and accessible to diagnosis and early removal. So why wait? The above arguments justify RFA for NDBE at least in the setting of controlled trials at specialized centers. As listed in Table 5.1, persons <50 years of age [33] with symptomatic NDBE and positive family history for gastrointestinal cancer should be recommended to undergo RFA. Contraindications against RFA are listed in Table 5.2.

5.8 Radiofrequency Ablation and Antireflux Surgery

GERD is a life style disease with impaired function of the antireflux mechanism of the esophagus [34]. Effective antireflux surgery restores the geometry and length of the high-pressure zone at the esophagogastric junction to eliminate GERD symptoms and gastroesophageal reflux, as assessed by quality of life assessment and impedance-pH monitoring (reflux monitoring), respectively [10, 35]. In contrast to this, medical therapy acts by altering the pH of the reflux without attenuating the reflux *per se* [6, 7]. In addition to bile gastric acid, duodenal bile salts and pancreatic enzymes are reported to contribute to the development of dysplasia and cancer within the columnar lined esophagus [1, 8, 9, 20]. PPI therapy alkalinizes the reflux [6], which is suggested to foster the cancerogenic effect of the bile salts and pancreatic enzymes and thus seems to trigger the events leading to the development of NDBE, dysplasia and cancer [1, 8, 9, 20]. In line with this notion, patients with a history of proton pump inhibitor therapy had a 3.5-fold increased risk for the development of esophageal adenocarcinoma compared to those who did not [36]. An increasing body of evidence indicates that antireflux surgery may foster the regression of Barrett's esophagus. Mabrut et al. [37], Gurksi et al. [38] and Csendes et al. [39] demonstrated that Barrett's esophagus regresses after effective antireflux surgery. Zaninotto et al. [14] recently compared the impact of medical vs. surgical therapy on the histopathology and genetics of Barrett's esophagus after 5 years. When compared to medical therapy, antireflux surgery was more effective in promoting regression and reversal of the genetic abnormalities (CDX2 expression) within short segment Barrett's esophagus [14]. Both forms of therapy did not affect long segment Barrett's esophagus. A recent meta-analysis indicated that, when compared to medical therapy, antireflux surgery is more effective to prevent the progression of NDBE towards dysplasia and cancer, and to favor regression of NDBE, but both types of therapies could not prevent the development of cancer [40]. Lagergren et al. [41] recently demonstrated that antireflux surgery could not prevent cancer development. As a major drawback, this study did not differentiate between effective and failed fundoplications and the pre-operative histopathology in all cases. Taken together, effective antireflux surgery seems capable of altering the destiny of CLE. Therefore it seems justified to question if antireflux surgery contributes to increase the yield of RFA for the elimination of NDBE (Fig. 5.5).

Hubbard and Velanovich [42] examined the feasibility of RFA after effective fundoplication in persons with NDBE. Three months after RFA NDBE was eliminated in six out of seven patients, one patient required an additional RFA for the removal of recurrent Barrett's esophagus.

In a retrospective study dos Santos et al. [43] included 14 patients with symptomatic GERD (partially responding to PPI therapy) and CLE (NDBE, $n=11$; low-grade dysplasia, $n=1$). Following RFA treatment for the eradication of the CLE, the patients underwent fundoplication for the elimination of their GERD symptoms; follow up was for 17 months (range 3–33 months). After two (range 1–6) RFA treatments all patients were free of NDBE and dysplasia. Eleven and three patients underwent laparoscopic and endoscopic fundoplication, respectively. Fundoplications were conducted 6 weeks after the first or second RFA session; in four patients the authors performed RFA before and after fundoplication. There were no complications after RFA, while two patients had complications after fundoplications (atrial fibrillation, pneumonia).

O'Connell and Velanovich [44] compared the effect of RFA and proton pump inhibitor therapy ($n=28$) versus RFA during ($n=10$) or 3 months before ($n=7$) and after ($n=2$) laparoscopic fundoplication for the elimination of NDBE (total 19 patients in the RFA + surgery group). Mean length of NDBE was similar in both groups (p = NS). After 1 year follow up NDBE was eliminated in 94.2 vs. 75.0 %, in patients undergoing RFA + fundoplication vs. RFA + proton pump inhibitor therapy, respectively. Complications did not occur.

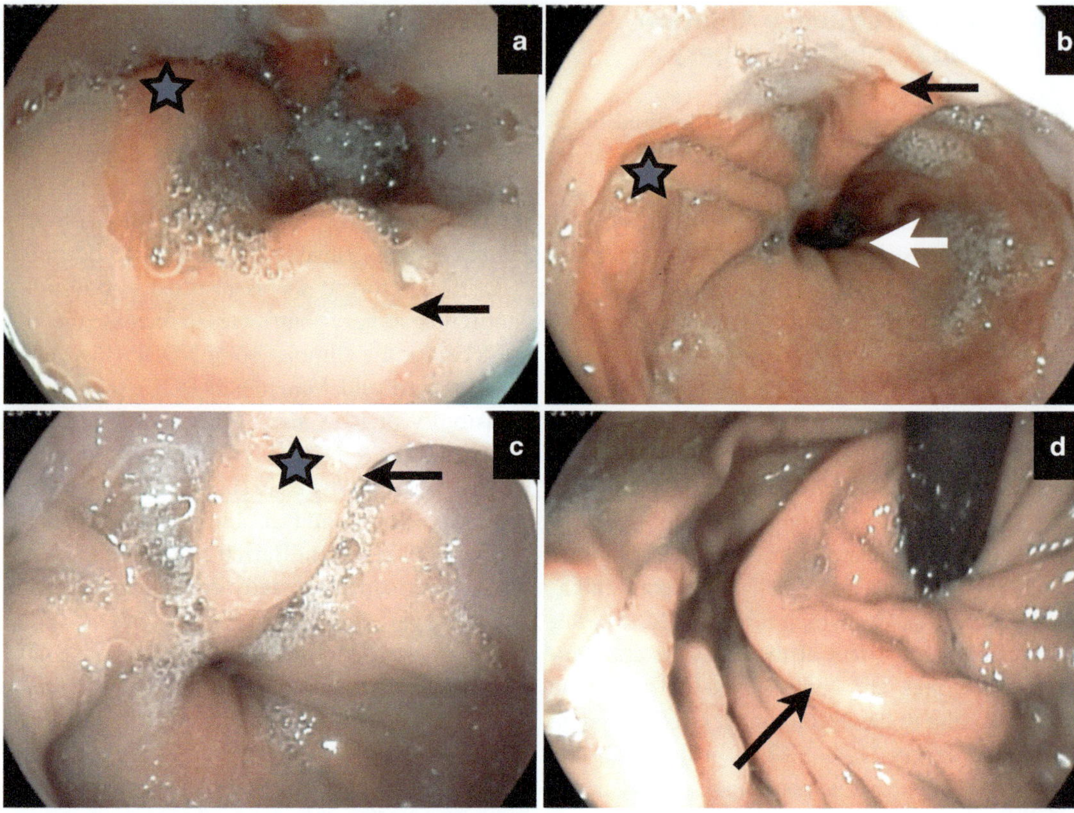

Fig. 5.5 Antegrade endoscopic images before (**a**, **b**) and after (**c**, **d**) radiofrequency ablation (*RFA*) and fundoplication for treatment of symptomatic non-dysplastic Barrett's esophagus in a 38 year-old male (4 months interval between RFA and fundoplication, images obtained 2 weeks before RFA and 6 months after fundoplication). (**a**, **b**) *Pre-RFA* endoscopic image of the irregular squamocolumnar junction with minimal (**a**) and maximal air insufflation (**b**), *arrows* mark the irregular squamocolumnar junction (*SCJ*) – note the proximal dislocation of the SCJ during air insufflation (*asterisk* marks start of gastric type fold), (**c**) antegrade endoscopy of the regular SCJ after RFA and fundoplication (*arrow*), (**d**) retrograde view towards the fundic wrap around the esophagogastric junction (*black arrow* in d marks the lower limit of the impression caused by the fundic wrap). SCJ-histopatholgy after fundoplication revealed cardiac and oxyntocardiac mucosa with absence of goblet cells

Goers et al. [45] recently tested the effect of concomitant RFA during laparoscopic fundoplication for the treatment of NDBE. The study included ten patients with 17 months follow up. Elimination of NDBE was achieved in 60 and 90 % of the patients after the 1st and 3rd RFA session, respectively. All patients showed a normal endoscopic appearance (Hill grade I). All eight patients undergoing postoperative esophageal manometry and reflux monitoring showed normal findings. Major complications in two patients included one stricture and one perforation within the RFA-treated segment. The management of the complications is not reported in the paper. Taken together, the above data indicate that effective antireflux surgery contributes to increase the yield of RFA for the elimination of NDBE.

In line with the observations made about the treatment of dysplasia and early cancer, the number of RFA treatments required for the complete eradication of NDBE increases with the length of endoscopically visible CLE (up to six sessions) and the size of the hiatal hernia [42–46].

Taken together, the published evidence justifies the combination of RFA and antireflux surgery for the management of symptomatic NDBE within prospective studies. Future trials should address if RFA should be conducted before, during or after antireflux surgery and which type of antireflux

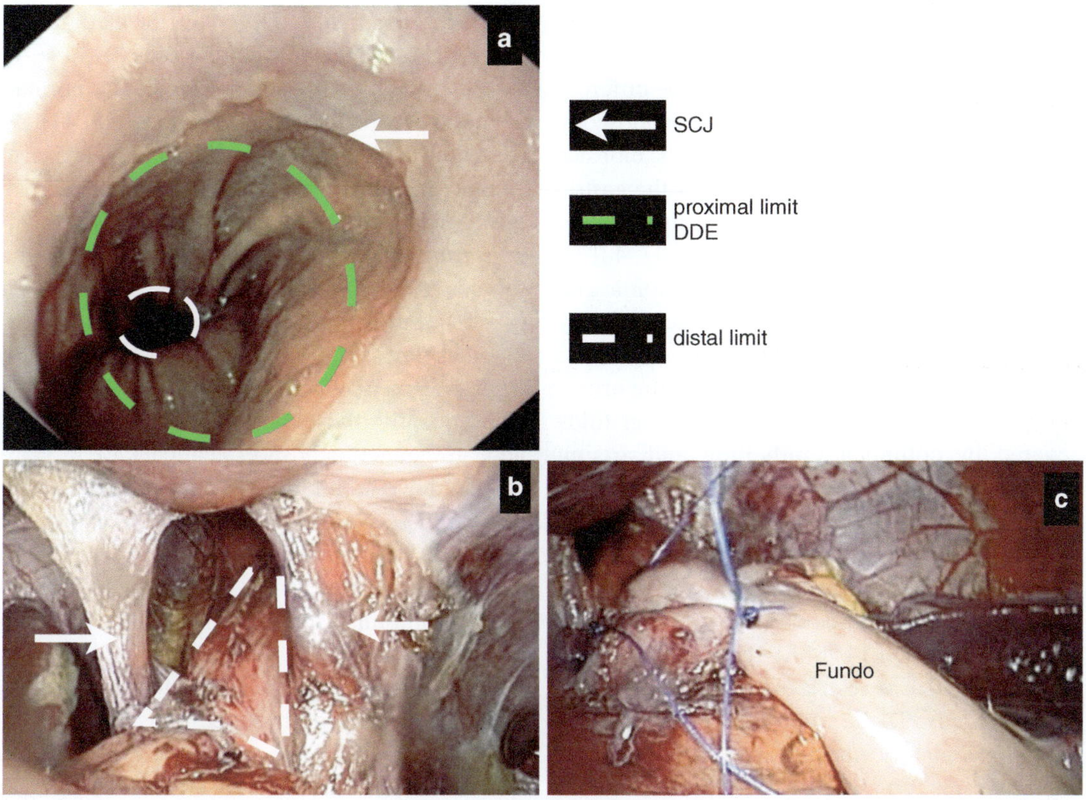

Fig. 5.6 Antegrade endoscopy (**a**) and laparoscopy (**b**, **c**) of the dilated distal esophagus (DDE). (**a**) Proximal (*green line*) and distal limit (*white line*) of the DDE: this is the reflux-damaged, fold forming dilated esophagus lined by a columnar epithelium, as described in the text. The squamooxyntic gap equals the distance between the squamocolumnar junction (*SCJ*) and the distal limit of the DDE (*white line*). (**b**) Laparoscopic view towards the esophageal hiatus (*arrows* mark the diaphragmatic crura). The *dotted white line* marks the DDE, which is included in the fundic wrap during the fundoplication (**c**) (DDE and squamooxyntic gap according to refs. ([47, 48])

procedure should be offered (laparoscopic vs. endoscopic fundoplication, magnetic sphincter).

5.9 The *Cardia*: Relevance for Diagnosis and Treatment

Recent evidence indicates that what has been taken as "gastric" cardia in fact represents the *dilated distal esophagus* (DDE) [47] (Fig. 5.6). Due to gastroesophageal reflux the distal portion of the esophagus gets damaged, dilated and forms mucosal folds covered by a columnar epithelium [34, 47]. Thus the *dilated distal esophagus* is mistaken as proximal stomach during the endoscopy, i.e. the so-called rugal folds, where *ruga* (latin) and *fold* (English) signify the same thing [18] (Fig. 5.6a).

According to a novel understanding the *dilated distal esophagus* represents the earliest morphologic consequence of GERD and precedes the stage of the disease where CLE becomes visible during endoscopy [47].

During over-eating the gastric distention propagates and dilates the distal esophagus [34, 47], which gets exposed to the gastric content. Initially the esophageal dilations are transient, and become permanent over time [34]. At this stage the distal, infra-diaphragmatic portion of the esophagus is almost permanently exposed to the reflux. This in turn fosters the inflammation-induced replacement of the squamous epithelium by CLE (±IM, intestinal metaplasia) and concomitant damage of the lower esophageal sphincter [34, 47]. Over time the process extends proximally towards and above the level of the diaphragm. Due to the fact that the mucosa of the reflux-damaged distal esophagus is dilated, folded and covered by a columnar epithelium (CLE) it cannot be differentiated from the proximal stomach by endoscopy [18, 47, 48]. However, in GERD patients, biopsies obtained from the proximal portion of the gastric type folds contain CLE, and not the oxyntic mucosa of the proximal stomach [4, 5, 47, 48].

Based on the works of Chandrasoma and DeMeester [47, 48], the endoscopic anatomy of the esophagogastric junction needs to be revised (Fig. 5.5). In GERD patients, the proximal portion of the longitudinal mucosal folds covered by columnar epithelium and arising circumferentially at the distal limit of the tubular esophagus (the so-called gastric type folds) contain CLE. Thus, in GERD patients, the cardia represents the *dilated distal esophagus* and does not contain the oxyntic mucosa of the proximal stomach [47]. At the early stage of GERD, the CLE is restricted to the *dilated distal esophagus* (DDE), which extends distal to an endoscopically normal appearing squamo-columnar junction. At an advanced stage of the disease the squamo-columnar junction becomes irregular: tongues, segments and islands of columnar lining become visible during endoscopy [48] (Fig. 5.6a). Conceptually, the entire distance between the proximal limit of the squamo-columnar junction (SCJ) and the biopsy level that contains the transition between CLE and gastric oxyntic mucosa defines the length of the so-called squamo-oxyntic gap [48] (Fig. 5.6a). The fusion of biopsy level information and the respective histopathology (CM, OCM, oxyntic mucosa) makes it possible to assess the dimensions of the gap and the DDE [47, 48]. The distance between the proximal and distal biopsy level within the endoscopically visible gastric type folds containing CLE defines the length of the dilated distal esophagus [47] (Fig. 5.6a). Thus the dimensions of the dilated distal esophagus cannot be assessed by endoscopy and require the histopathology of measured multi level biopsies obtained from the endoscopically visible esophagogastric junction. The relevance of the dilated distal esophagus for diagnosis, RFA and surgery remains to be established.

The *dilated distal esophagus* (the cardia) contains intestinal metaplasia (IM) in 20–30 % of GERD patients with an endoscopically normal-appearing esophagogastric junction [4, 5, 47]. As the endoscopically visible NDBE gives rise to adenocarcinoma of the so-called tubular esophagus (AEG I), NDBE at an endoscopically normal-appearing esophagogastric junction may progress towards adenocarcinoma of the cardia (AEG II or III) [49, 50]. Furthermore, the majority of adenocarcinomas develop within the mid to distal third of a given segment of columnar lined esophagus [51]. Consequently those with NDBE at a normal appearing junction or short segment CLE (≤3 cm) harbor the risk for cancer development within their *dilated distal esophagus* (carcinoma of the cardia). Therefore the *dilated distal esophagus* should be included in the diagnosis (multi level biopsy sampling) for exclusion of NDBE, dysplasia and cancer.

In addition, the proximal portion of the endoscopically visible gastric type folds (i.e. the cardia) contains CLE [4, 47]. Consequently RFA should include the proximal 1–3 cm (=treatment length of the HALO^{360} balloon) of the cardia, irrespective of the presence or absence of endoscopically visible NDBE to eliminate the risk of NDBE and cancer formation within the *dilated distal esophagus*. Therefore, after successful eradication of CLE of the cardia the post RFA endoscopy will show squamous lined esophagus below the level of the diaphragmatic hiatus (i.e. the abdominal portion of the esophagus is resealed by a squamous epithelium).

Inasmuch antireflux surgery should target the dilated distal esophagus (i.e. enwrap the dilated distal esophagus, the dimension of which is assessed by preoperative multi level biopsies from the cardia) is currently under investigation (Fig. 5.6b, c).

5.10 Asymptomatic Non-dysplastic Barrett's Esophagus

As a matter of fact, 40–70 % of esophageal adenocarcinomas develop without a preceding history of GERD symptoms [36]. A meta-analysis demonstrated that less than 5 % of all adenocarcinomas are assessed during surveillance of

Barrett's esophagus [13, 15]. In addition, the detection of esophageal adenocarcinoma during surveillance of Barrett's esophagus is associated with a lower tumor stage at the time of diagnosis and a longer survival [52]. Large population based studies found that esophageal adenocarcinomas detected during surveillance of Barrett's esophagus account for less than 10 % of all cancers registered during the same time period [53]. Currently screening and surveillance exclude those without symptoms [13] and thus fail to detect asymptomatic Barrett's esophagus [54, 55]. This explains why we still miss more than 90 % of the cancers at an earlier stage and why current surveillance strategies fail to counteract cancer development [53].

Prospective studies should examine the impact of screening for asymptomatic Barrett's esophagus. Recent studies indicate that this may be effective for both genders at an age of 50 years [56]. Due to the positive associations between colonic disorders and asymptomatic NDBE in 25 % of cases [55], screening endoscopy of the esophagus should be combined with ano-recto-colonoscopy.

The above considerations indicate that *asymptomatic* NDBE seems to be at least at similar risk for cancer development compared to symptomatic NDBE [13, 15, 52]. Consequently it seems justified to consider the ablation of asymptomatic NDBE in the setting of a prospective study. Future trials will have to examine if RFA of asymptomatic NDBE should be followed by an antireflux procedure (fundoplication, magnetic sphincter) [42–46, 57].

5.11 Summary

Non-dysplastic Barrett's esophagus offers the unique and promising opportunity to stop the progression towards dysplasia and cancer before it becomes dangerous for the patient and difficult for the physician. The combination of RFA with antireflux surgery seems to increase the success rate of ablation and may be of relevance for cancer prevention. Future studies should examine the durability of RFA and fundoplication for cancer prevention. Finally we have to assess the impact of RFA on the elimination of asymptomatic NDBE and to what extent this contributes to cancer prevention. The time seems ready for an "act" instead of "wait and see" policy in the management of NDBE. The tables are turning and we need to keep our minds open and act before cancer develops.

Key Points

- Symptomatic non-dysplastic Barrett's esophagus (NDBE) results from gastroesophageal reflux and harbors a 0.5 % annual risk for cancer development, the same risk as a colon polyp
- Causal management would include the elimination of metaplasia and reflux
- The genetic characteristics of NDBE are similar to dysplasia and cancer. Diagnostic (biopsy sampling error) and molecular characteristics of NDBE are similar to dysplasia and cancer
- Radiofrequency ablation (RFA) is safe, effective and durable
- Effective antireflux surgery increases the yield of RFA for the elimination of NDBE
- Forty to seventy percent of esophageal adenocarcinomas develop *without* preceding symptoms of gastroesophageal reflux disease (GERD) and less than 10 % of cancers are detected via screening and surveillance of symptomatic NDBE
- Future trials should assess if screening, surveillance and ablation of *asymptomatic* Barrett's esophagus may be beneficial for cancer prevention

References

1. Spechler SJ, Fitzgerald RC, Prasad GA, Wang KK (2010) History, molecular mechanism, and endoscopic treatment of Barrett's esophagus. Gastroenterology 138(3):854–869
2. Mueller J, Werner M, Stolte M (2004) Barrett's esophagus: histopathologic definitions and diagnostic criteria. World J Surg 28(2):148–154
3. Chandrasoma P, Wijetunge S, DeMeester S et al (2012) Columnar-lined esophagus without intestinal metaplasia has no proven risk of adenocarcinoma. Am J Surg Pathol 36(1):1–7

4. Ringhofer C, Lenglinger J, Izay B et al (2008) Histopathology of the endoscopic esophagogastric junction in patients with gastroesophageal reflux disease. Wien Klin Wochenschr 120(11):350–359
5. Lenglinger J, Izay B, Eisler M et al (2009) Barrett's esophagus: size of the problem and diagnostic value of a novel histopathology classification. Eur Surg 41(1):26–39
6. Triadafilopoulos G (2008) Proton pump inhibitor in Barrett's esophagus: pluripotent but controversial. Eur Surg 40(2):58–65
7. Tamhankar AP, Peters JH, Portale G et al (2004) Omeprazole does not reduce gastroesophageal reflux: new insights using multichannel intraluminal impedance technology. J Gastrointest Surg 8(7):890–897
8. Theisen J, Peters JH, Fein M et al (2005) The mutagenic potential of duodenoesophageal reflux. Ann Surg 241:63–68
9. Fein M, Peters JH, DeMeester TR (2007) Carcinogenesis in reflux disease: in search for bile-specific effects. Microsurgery 27(8):647–650
10. Koch OO, Kaindlsdorfer A, Antoniou SA et al (2012) Laparoscopic Nissen versus Toupet fundoplication: objective and subjective results of a prospective randomized trail. Surg Endosc 26(2):413–422, Epub 2011 Sep 5
11. Vallböhmer D, DeMeester SR, Oh DS et al (2006) Antireflux surgery normalizes cyclooxygenase-2 expression in squamous epithelium of the distal esophagus. Am J Gastroenterol 101(7):1458–1466
12. Fleischer DE, Odze R, Overholt BF et al (2010) The case for endoscopic treatment of non-dysplastic and low grade dysplastic Barrett's esophagus. Dig Dis Sci 55:1918–1931
13. Spechler SJ (2007) Screening and surveillance for Barrett's esophagus – an unresolved dilemma. Nat Clin Pract Gastroenterol Hepatol 4(9):470–471
14. Zaninotto G, Parente P, Salvador R et al (2012) Long term follow up of Barrett's epithelium: medical versus antireflux surgical therapy. J Gastrointest Surg 16(1): 7–14; discussion 14–15. Epub 2011 Nov 16
15. Dulai GS, Guha S, Kahn KL et al (2002) Preoperative prevalence of Barrett's esophagus in esophageal adenocarcinomas: a systematic review. Gastroenterology 122:26–33
16. Rieder F, Biancani P, Harnett K et al (2010) Inflammatory mediators in gastroesophageal reflux disease: impact on esophageal motility, fibrosis, and carcinogenesis. Am J Physiol 298:G571–G581
17. Chandrasoma PT (2006) Columnar lined esophagus: what it is and what it tells us. Eur Surg 38(3):197–209
18. Lenglinger J, Eisler M, Wrba F et al (2008) Update: histopathology-based definition of gastroesophageal reflux disease and Barrett's esophagus. Eur Surg 40(4): 165–175
19. Castillo D, Puig S, Iglesias M et al (2012) Activation of the BMP-4 pathway and the early expression of CDX2 characterize non-specialized columnar metaplasia in a human model of Barrett's esophagus. J Gastrointest Surg 16(2):227–237; discussion 237. Epub 2011 Nov 11
20. Huo X, Zhang HY, Zhang XI et al (2010) Acid and bile salt-induced CDX2 expression differs in esophageal squamous cells from patients with and without Barrett's esophagus. Gastroenterology 139(1):194–203
21. Arora G, Basra S, Roorda AK, Triadafilopoulos G (2009) Radiofrequency ablation for Barrett's esophagus. Eur Surg 41/1:19–25
22. Shaheen NJ, Sharma P, Overholt BF et al (2009) Radiofrequency ablation in Barrett's esophagus with dysplasia. N Engl J Med 360:2277–2288
23. Shaheen NJ, Overholt BF, Sampliner RE et al (2011) Durability of radiofrequency ablation in Barrett's esophagus with dysplasia. Gastroenterology 141:460–468
24. Fleischer DE, Overholt BF, Sharma VK et al (2008) Endoscopic ablation of Barrett's esophagus: a multicenter study with 2.5-year follow up. Gastrointest Endosc 68(5):867–876
25. Lyday WD, Corbett FS, Kuperman DA et al (2010) Radiofrequency ablation of Barrett's esophagus: outcomes of 429 patients from a multicenter community practice registry. Endoscopy 42:272–278
26. Fleischer DE, Overholt BF, Sharma VK et al (2010) Endoscopic radiofrequency ablation for Barrett's esophagus: 5-year outcomes from a prospective multicenter trial. Endoscopy 42(10):781–789
27. Pouw RE, Gondrie JJ, Rygiel AM et al (2009) Properties of the neosquamous epithelium after radiofrequency ablation of Barrett's esophagus containing neoplasia. Am J Gastroenterol 104(6):1366–1373
28. Beaumont H, Gondrie JJ, McMahon BP et al (2009) Stepwise radiofrequency ablation of Barrett's esophagus rpeserves esophageal inner diameter, compliance, and motility. Endoscopy 41(1):2–8
29. Inadomi JM, Somsouk M, Madanick RD et al (2009) A cost-utility analysis of ablative therapy for Barrett's esophagus. Gastroenterology 136(7):2101–2114
30. Gray NA, Odze RD, Spechler SJ (2011) Buried metaplasia after endoscopic ablation of Barrett's esophagus: a systematic review. Am J Gastroenterol 106(11): 1899–1908
31. Wani S, Puli SR, Shaheen NJ et al (2009) Esophageal adenocarcinoma in Barrett's esophagus after endoscopic ablative therapy: a meta-analysis and systemic review. Am J Gastroenterol 104:502–513
32. Takubo K, Aida J, Naomoto Y et al (2009) Cardiac rather than intestinal type background in endoscopic resection specimens of minute Barrett adenocarcinoma. Hum Pathol 40(1):65–74
33. Rubenstein JH, Scheiman JM, Sadeghi S et al (2011) Esophageal adenocarcinoma incidence in individuals with gastroesophageal reflux: synthesis and estimates from population studies. Am J Gastroenterol 106(2): 254–260
34. Ayazi SH, Tamhankar A, DeMeester SR et al (2010) The impact of gastric distension on the lower esophageal sphincter and its exposure to acid gastric juice. Ann Surg 252(1):57–62

35. Lord RVN, DeMeester SR, Peters JH et al (2009) Hiatal hernia, lower esophageal sphincter incometence, and effectiveness of Nissen fundoplciation in the spectrum of gastroesophageal reflux disease. J Gastrointest Surg 13(4):602–610
36. Lagergren J, Bergström R, Lindgren A et al (1999) Symptomatic gastroesophageal reflux as a risk factor for esophageal adenocarcinoma. N Eng J Med 340(11): 825–831
37. Mabrut JY, Baulieux J, Adham M et al (2003) Impact of antireflux operation on columnar lined esophagus. J Am Coll Surg 196(1):60–67
38. Gurski RR, Peters JH, Hagen JA et al (2003) Barrett's esophagus can and does regress after antireflux surgery: a study of prevalence and predictive features. J Am Coll Surg 196(5):706–712
39. Csendes A, Braghetto I, Burdiles P et al (2009) Late results of the surgical treatment of 125 patients with short-segment Barrett esophagus. Arch Surg 144(10): 921–927
40. Chang EY, Morris CD, Seltman AK et al (2007) The effect of antireflux surgery on esophageal carcinogenesis in patients with Barrett esophagus: a systematic review. Ann Surg 246(1):11–21
41. Lagergren J, Ye W, Lagegren P, Lu Y (2010) The risk of esophageal adenocarcinoma after antireflux surgery. Gastroenterology 138(4):1297–1301
42. Hubbard N, Velanovich V (2007) Endoscopic endoluminal radiofrequency ablation of Barrett's esophagus in patients with fundoplication. Surg Endosc 21:625–628
43. dos Santos RS, Bizekis C, Ebright M et al (2010) Radiofrequency ablation fro Barrett's esophagus and low grade dysplasia in combination with antireflux procedure: a new paradigm. J Thorac Cardiovasc Surg 139(3):713–716
44. O'Connell K, Velanovich V (2011) Effects of Nissen fundplication on endoscopic endoluminal radiofrequency ablation of Barrett's esophagus. Surg Endosc 25(3):830–834
45. Goers TA, Leao P, Cassera MA et al (2011) Concomitant endoscopic radiofrequency ablation and laparoscopic reflux operative results in more effective and efficient treatment of Barrett's esophagus. J Am Coll Surg 213(4):486–492
46. Korst RJ, Santana-Joseph S, Rutledge JR et al (2011) Effect of hiatal hernia size and columnar segment length on the success of radiofrequency ablation for Barrett's esophagus: a single-center, phase II clinical trial. J Thorac Cardiovasc Surg 142(2):1168–1173
47. Chandrasoma P, Wijetunge S, Ma Y, DeMeester S et al (2011) The dilated distal esophagus: a new entity that is the pathologic basis of early gastroesophageal reflux disease. Am J Surg Pathol 35(12):1873–1881
48. Chandrasoma P, Wijetunge S, DeMeester SR et al (2010) The histologic squamo-oxyntic gap: an accurate and reproducible diagnostic marker of gastroesophageal reflux disease. Am J Surg Pathol 34(11): 1574–1581
49. Wijetunge S, Ma Y, DeMeester S et al (2010) Association of adenocarcinoma of the distal esophagus, "gastroesophageal junction", and "gastric cardia" with gastric pathology. Am J Surg Pathol 34(10):1521–1527
50. Siewert JR, Stein HJ, Feith M (2006) Adenocarcinoma of the esophago-gastric junction. Scand J Surg 95(4):260–269
51. Theisen J, Stein HJ, Feith M et al (2006) Preferred location for the development of esophageal adenocarcinoma within a segment of intestinal metaplasia. Surg Endosc 20(2):235–238
52. Corley DA, Levin TR, Habel LA et al (2002) Surveillance and survival in Barrett's adenocarcinomas: a population based study. Gastroenterology 122:633–640
53. Hvid-Jensen F, Pedersen L, Mohr Drewes A et al (2011) Incidence of adenocarcinoma among patients with Barrett's esophagus. N Engl J Med 365:1375–1383
54. Gerson LB, Shetler K, Triadafilopoulos G (2002) Prevalence of Barrett's esophagus in asymptomatic individuals. Gastroenterology 123:461–467
55. Rex DK, Cummings OW, Shaw M (2003) Screening for Barrett's esophagus in colonoscopy patients with and without heartburn. Gastroenterology 125:1670–1677
56. Rubenstein JH, Mattek N, Eisen G (2010) Age- and sex-specific yield of Barrett's esophagus by endoscopy indication. Gastrointest Endosc 71(1):21–27
57. Bonavina L, DeMeester T, Fockens P et al (2010) Laparoscopic sphincter augmentation device eliminates reflux symptoms and normalizes esophageal acid exposure. Ann Surg 252(5):857–862

Esophageal Preservation in Barrett's Esophagus with High-Grade Dysplasia and Mucosal Adenocarcinoma

6

Thomas J. Watson and Jeffrey H. Peters

6.1 Introduction

A surgeon may witness a radical shift in therapies a few times during a career. For example, the introduction and refinement of laparoscopic and thoracoscopic techniques have brought about a revolution in the management of a multitude of abdominal and thoracic disease processes over the past generation. Another more recent, yet equally significant, paradigm shift has been the popularization of endoscopic therapies for early esophageal neoplasia. Conditions such as Barrett's esophagus (BE) with high-grade dysplasia (HGD) or intramucosal adenocarcinoma (IMC), which were generally treated by esophagectomy just a few years ago, are now treated by endoscopic techniques in the majority of cases. In fact, recent guidelines proposed by the American Gastroenterological Association recommend endoscopic resection and ablation as the procedures of choice for early esophageal neoplasia in most patients [1]. Due to the availability and popularization of such efficacious and low-risk endoscopic therapies, many individuals previously referred for surgery are now spared from esophageal resection and reconstruction, with their inherent morbidity, potential for mortality, and negative impact on alimentary function.

6.2 State of the Art: Esophagectomy for Early Esophageal Neoplasia

With such a rapid change in therapeutic paradigms, the treating physician must be knowledgeable about the indications for, and outcomes following, esophagectomy for early esophageal neoplasia so as to have a basis against which endoscopic alternatives may be compared. Esophagectomy has been the prevailing standard of care for most cases of early esophageal neoplasia for decades, with a well-established track record in terms of cure rates, perioperative morbidity and mortality, and long-term quality of life.

The rationale for esophageal resection in cases of BE with HGD has been based on two factors: (1) occult carcinoma has been found in a significant fraction of esophagectomy specimens, averaging approximately 37 % in multiple large surgical series, even when a thorough preoperative biopsy protocol failed to detect invasion [2]; and (2) invasive cancer may arise within dysplastic BE over the short to medium term if the esophagus is left in place [3]. Esophagectomy,

T.J. Watson (✉) • J.H. Peters
Division of Thoracic and Foregut Surgery,
Department of Surgery,
University of Rochester School of Medicine and Dentistry, 601 Elmwood Avenue, Box Surgery,
Rochester, NY 14642, USA
e-mail: thomas_watson@urmc.rochester.edu

L. Bonavina (ed.), *Innovation in Esophageal Surgery*,
DOI 10.1007/978-88-470-2469-4_6,

Fig. 6.1 Esophagectomy options. The operation should be tailored to the characteristics of the patient and the disease process

Less invasive ↓ **More Invasive**

- "Minimally invasive"
- Transhiatal with cervical esophagogastrostomy+/-vagal-sparing
- Laparotomy with jejunal interposition
- Right thoracotomy, laparotomy, intrathoracic esophagogastrostomy
- Right thoracotomy, laparotomy, cervical esophagogastrostomy
- Left thoracotomy/thoracoabdominal with intrathoracic esophagogastrostomy
- Radical (en bloc)
  - with 2-field lymphadenectomy
  - with 3-field lymphadenectomy
  - using gastric pull-up
  - using colon or jejunal interposition

therefore, is both curative and prophylactic. An advantage of esophagectomy is that the entire region of neoplasia, and mucosa at risk for development of subsequent neoplasia, is removed in a single therapeutic session; it is the ultimate total ablation technique. Critics of esophageal resection in this circumstance, however, have considered esophagectomy "radical prophylaxis" for a microscopic disease process [4]. Citing reported perioperative morbidity and mortality rates, as well as potential adverse effects on long-term quality of life following esophagectomy, such authors recommend caution when considering surgical intervention for a condition that may be pre-malignant.

Large population-based studies have shown significant mortality when esophagectomy is performed for cancer. In a report from 2003 describing the experience in U.S. Veterans Administration hospitals from 1991 to 2000, 30-day postoperative mortality in 1,777 esophagectomies performed in 109 facilities was 9.8 % [5]. Most operations, however, were undertaken in low-volume institutions, as only 1.6 esophagectomies were done per year in the average facility. A publication from 2007 utilized the Nationwide Inpatient Sample to assess esophagectomy outcomes in 17,395 patients over the years 1999–2003 [6]. Overall mortality was 8.7 %, with high-volume centers obtaining significantly lower rates compared to low-volume institutions. In specialty centers, contemporary data derived from the U.S. and Europe show far better rates of perioperative mortality following esophagectomy for cancer, in the range of 3–5 % [7–10]. Such data are commonly quoted by gastroenterologists and surgeons when discussing esophagectomy as an alternative for BE with HGD or IMC.

More relevant, however, are data specific to esophagectomy for early neoplasia. A literature review published in 2007 detailed the reported experience with esophagectomy for HGD over the 20-year period from 1987 to 2007 [2]. In 22 studies covering 530 patients, the overall perioperative mortality was 0.94 %, representing only five total deaths. No report included more than one death and 17 of the 22 studies included no mortalities. A number of plausible factors may explain the lower mortality when esophagectomy is undertaken for HGD as compared to more advanced malignancy, including patient selection, lack of dysphagia and weight loss, absence of preoperative chemotherapy and radiation, less invasive surgical approaches, and the fact that the reported outcomes are predominantly from specialty centers. When discussing esophagectomy as a treatment option for early esophageal neoplasia, a 1 % chance of perioperative mortality appears to be the appropriate rate to quote from the literature, assuming a good risk patient and an expert surgical team. Since data regarding endoscopic therapies also are derived from specialty centers, such surgical outcomes are the appropriate comparators.

Experienced esophageal surgeons should possess a multitude of operative approaches and techniques for esophagectomy in their therapeutic armamentarium (Fig. 6.1); a "one size fits all" mind set is not appropriate. The procedure selected for a particular individual may depend upon a variety of patient factors as well as surgeon biases and preferences.

When operation is undertaken for locoregionally-advanced cancer, a thorough lymphadenectomy becomes an important component of the procedure. Many surgeons opt in such cases to perform a combined thoracic and abdominal (two-field) or thoracic, abdominal and cervical (three-field) lymphadenectomy. The thoracic component of the lymph node dissection requires a thoracotomy, thoracoabdominal incision or thoracoscopy for access. For cases of neoplasia confined to the epithelium or mucosa where the potential for nodal spread is low, the need for lymphadenectomy is obviated, permitting elimination of thoracic incisions altogether. As transthoracic esophagectomy has been shown to be associated with a higher rate of postoperative pulmonary complications compared to transhiatal resection [10], not to mention the potential for both short-term and long-term incisional pain, the avoidance of a thoracotomy is desirable when operation is undertaken for BE with HGD or IMC. A transhiatal esophagectomy (THE) without thoracotomy, or minimally invasive esophagectomy (MIE) via combined thoracoscopy and laparoscopy [11], should be utilized in such cases of early neoplasia where the risk of nodal metastasis is low.

The omission of a lymphadenectomy also permits preservation of the vagus nerves. The vagi typically are removed at the time of esophagectomy to facilitate complete resection of both local tumor and regional nodal metastases. As many of the side effects following esophagectomy are thought to result from the associated vagotomy, the preservation of vagal innervation has important implications relative to the long-term functional outcomes after foregut resection and reconstruction. Vagal-sparing esophagectomy (VSE) has been shown to be associated with decreased perioperative morbidity, thought secondary to a lower incidence of sepsis, conduit ischemia and anastomotic leakage, as well as fewer long-term gastrointestinal side effects such as dumping, diarrhea, weight loss, and anastomotic stricture, relative to standard esophagectomy performed with vagal resection [12]. The esophageal surgeon is advised to consider these less invasive and morbid surgical approaches, such as THE, MIE or VSE, when operation is undertaken for early esophageal neoplasia in that long-term quality of life is an important consideration given the expectation of cure.

6.3 State of the Art: Endoscopic Therapies for Early Esophageal Neoplasia

6.3.1 Endoscopic Mucosal Resection

Initially described by surgeons in Japan for treatment of superficial squamous cell carcinoma of the esophagus [13], endoscopic mucosal resection (EMR) has been adopted by physicians in Europe and the US for excisional biopsy of small mucosal irregularities or discrete nodules in the setting of BE, as well as for potentially curative treatment of small foci of HGD or IMC. Two potential applications thus exist for EMR:

1. The resected specimen can serve as a wide and deep biopsy to guide subsequent definitive therapy (observation of non-neoplastic disease or esophagectomy for HGD/IMC with tailoring of the procedure based upon depth of tumor penetration);
2. The procedure can be performed with curative intent (with or without adjunctive mucosal ablation of residual non-nodular metaplasia/dysplasia) for tumors at low risk for metastatic spread to regional lymph nodes or distant sites.

As HGD or IMC are frequently multifocal in nature, EMR is typically used on endoscopically identifiable discrete nodules and combined with an ablative procedure to eliminate more widespread regions of synchronous microscopic neoplasia or metaplasia. Treatment adjuncts in such situations include radiofrequency (RF) ablation, cryotherapy, argon plasma coagulation (APC), multipolar electrocautery (MPEC) or photodynamic therapy (PDT). In contrast to ablation, EMR possesses the obvious advantage of providing a generous specimen for histologic assessment, including a determination of the presence of invasive carcinoma, the depth of invasion if present, the degree of differentiation of the tumor, the presence of lymphovascular invasion, and the freedom of disease at the lateral and deep resection margins. EMR improves the staging of early esophageal neoplasia compared to standard biopsy techniques and imaging modalities such as endoscopic ultrasonography.

Endoscopic therapies are appropriate with curative intent only when the neoplastic process appears to be limited to the mucosa and the potential for lymph node metastasis or systemic spread is low. Several series from the surgical literature have evaluated outcomes after esophagectomy with regional lymphadenectomy for esophageal adenocarcinoma and have correlated the incidence of nodal metastasis with the depth of tumor invasion. Tumors limited to the mucosa appear to have a limited potential for nodal disease, approximating 2–5 % [14–19]. For adenocarcinomas penetrating the muscularis mucosa and involving the submucosa, the incidence of nodal metastasis appears to increase significantly to around 25 %. Some series, however, would suggest that tumors invading into the superficial submucosa (SM1) have a low incidence of nodal metastasis, similar to disease limited to the mucosa, while deeper submucosal lesions portend a worse prognosis [15]. The validity of this observation, however, has been challenged by other studies [18, 19]. Tumors involving the muscularis propria have an even higher chance of associated nodal spread, in the range of 45–80 %. Thus, current opinion is that EMR is appropriate as therapy with curative intent only for tumors limited to the mucosa.

6.3.2 Endoscopic Mucosal Resection Techniques

A number of techniques have been described for performing EMR. All share the basic principle of identification of a defined segment of esophageal mucosa and excision using a snare cautery device. Differences in technique relate to the use of submucosal injection of saline (with or without dilute epinephrine) to separate the target lesion from the underlying muscle layer, and the manner in which the lesion is subsequently lifted and isolated for snare application. The term "endoscopic mucosal resection" is a misnomer in that the resection plane typically is within the submucosa, or at the interface of the submucosa and muscularis propria, and the resected specimen usually contains both mucosa and submucosa.

Perhaps the simplest variant of EMR is snare resection alone without elevation or submucosal injection. This technique is best applied to polypoid lesions of the esophageal mucosa, in that flat lesions cannot be snared without some form of mucosal elevation.

A common resection method has been the use of submucosal injection of saline with dilute epinephrine (10–20 mL injectate, 1:100,000 solution) to separate the mucosa from the underlying muscularis propria. The target lesion can then be aspirated into a specially designed cap (Olympus EMR-001, Olympus America, Center Valley, Pennsylvania, USA) attached to the end of a standard flexible adult endoscope ("cap-assisted" EMR.) The cap is equipped with an inner groove that allows seating of a standard cautery snare. Once the mucosa is within the cap, the snare can be tightened around the base of the lesion and cautery applied, amputating the specimen in the submucosal plane. Prior to application of cautery, the lesion should be gently "tugged" to give the operator a sense of mobility away from the muscularis and to prevent inadvertent full-thickness injury to the esophageal wall. The resected specimen typically remains within the cap and can be extracted as the endoscope is withdrawn.

A similar technique, and the one currently favored by the authors, is to use a variceal banding device with supplied cap system to isolate the target lesion. Various single-use multiband systems (Duette Multiband Mucosectomy System, Cook Medical, Bloomington, Indiana or Bard Six-Shooter, Bard Interventional Products, Billerica, Massachusetts, USA) are commercially available. The procedure involves suction of the mucosa into the cap (without prior submucosal injection) and application of a rubber band to the base of the elevated mucosa (Fig. 6.2), creating a pseudopolyp ("suck and ligate" EMR). The lesion is then excised either above or below the band using snare electrocautery (Fig. 6.3). An important principle underlying this technique is that the elasticity of the rubber band is not sufficient to hold the muscularis propria within

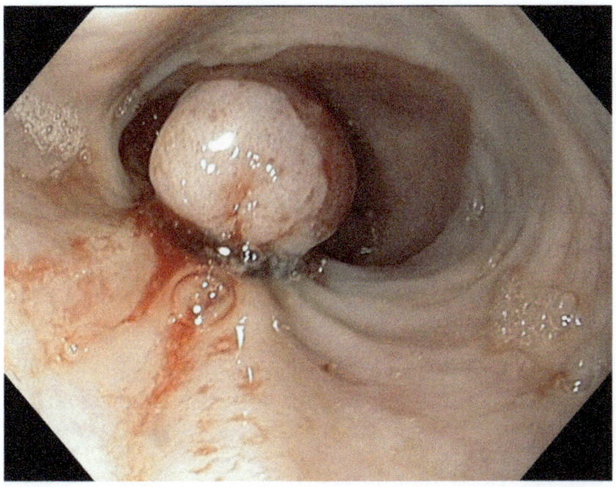

Fig. 6.2 "Suck and ligate" EMR utilizing a variceal band to create an esophageal mucosal pseudopolyp. An important principle behind this technique is that the band is not strong enough to hold the muscularis propria within it. Excision should remove only mucosa and submucosa

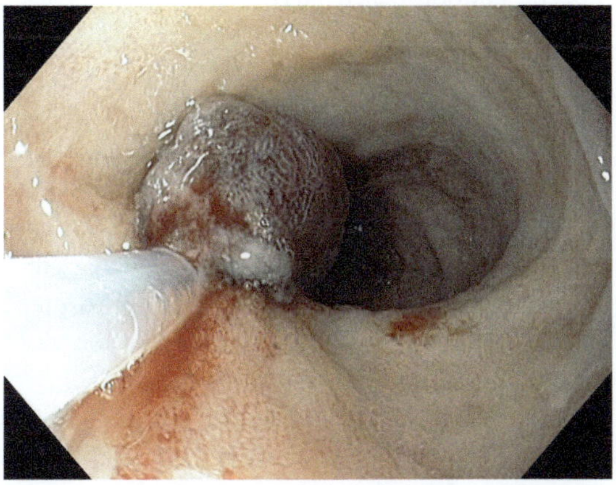

Fig. 6.3 Excision of the pseudopolyp using an electrocautery snare

it (Fig. 6.4). Excision of the pseudopolyp can proceed with confidence that a full-thickness perforation should not result. The excised specimen can be retrieved using any of a variety of devices such as a net or polypectomy grasper.

Advantages of this technique compared to cap-assisted resection are that submucosal injection is not necessary and that the snare does not need to be seated in the cap, a process that may be time-consuming and difficult to master. Disadvantages of the banding technique are the need to reintroduce the endoscope to pass/position the snare

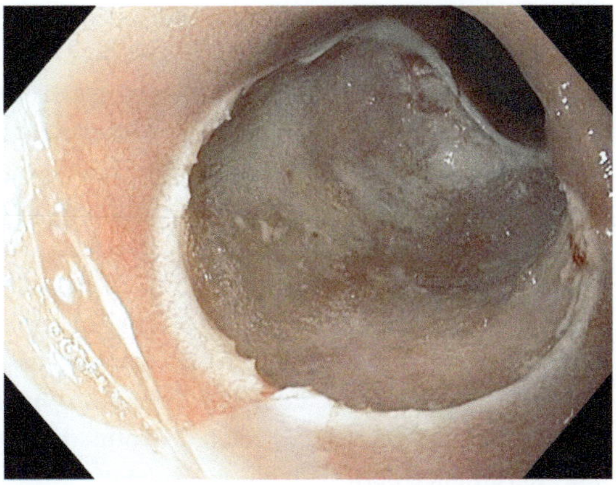

Fig. 6.4 Site of EMR. Note the plane of resection at the interface of the submucosa and muscularis propria

Table 6.1 Eligibility criteria for endoscopic mucosal resection (EMR)

1. No evidence of more advanced tumor (>T1), lymph node involvement or systemic metastasis on staging evaluation
2. Tumor deemed low-risk for lymphatic or systemic spread: (a) Lesion diameter <20 mm (b) Macroscopically polypoid or flat without ulceration (c) Well-differentiated or moderately differentiated adenocarcinoma (d) Limited to the mucosa on the basis of staging procedures (e.g. endoscopic ultrasound) and proven on histologic examination of resected specimen (e) No invasion of lymphatics or veins on histologic examination of resected specimen

and, again, to retrieve the excised specimen. A prospective, randomized trial demonstrated equivalency between "cap-assisted" EMR and "suck and ligate" EMR in terms of the maximum diameter of the resected specimen, the resection area and complication rates [20].

The largest experience with EMR for early esophageal adenocarcinoma was reported in 2007 by Ell et al. from Wiesbaden, Germany [21]. Their series included 100 patients from a total of 667 referred with suspected intraepithelial neoplasia. Eligibility criteria to undergo EMR are listed in Table 6.1. A total of 144 resections (1.47 per patient) were performed without major complications. Most tumors (69 %) occurred in the setting of short-segment BE. EMR was combined with either APC for short-segment BE or PDT for long-segment BE in 49 patients. Complete local remission was achieved in 99 out of the 100 patients in a mean of 1.9 months and with a maximum of three resections. Metachronous or recurrent disease occurred in 11 % of patients during a mean follow-up period of 36.7 months, though repeat treatment with EMR was successful in all cases. The calculated 5-year survival was 98 %, with no cancer-related deaths during the surveillance period.

A follow-up to this experience was published in 2008 [22]. The patient cohort had increased to 349 patients with a mean follow-up of 63.6 months. The majority of patients underwent EMR, though only 20 % had some form of mucosal ablation. Perhaps as a result of this low utilization of ablation, the metachronous neoplasia rate was up to 21.5 %. Despite this fact, the complete response rate was 97 % with only 3.7 % of patients requiring esophagectomy for failed endoscopic therapy. The 5-year survival was 84 % with no esophageal cancer-related deaths. These data underscore the feasibility of EMR in a highly select subgroup of patients referred with HGD or IMC and treated at a specialty center.

6.3.3 Mucosal Ablation

A number of mucosal ablative techniques also have been utilized as potentially curative treatments for esophageal metaplasia or early neoplasia. The nature of such therapies, however, is that the targeted epithelium is destroyed, making subsequent pathologic assessment and accurate staging impossible.

PDT and APC are the two endoscopic techniques most widely studied for ablation of residual metaplasia/dysplasia after EMR of focal lesions. Both procedures, however, have shortcomings in that multiple treatment sessions may be required, the depth of penetration is limited, complete elimination of pathologic mucosa is not guaranteed, buried BE under squamous epithelium has been observed, and a significant complication rate from esophageal strictures, perforations and photosensitivity (with PDT) has been reported.

Radiofrequency (RF) ablation recently has been introduced into practice and has the potential to avoid many of these limitations. Three RF devices, the HALO^{360}, HALO^{90}, and HALO^{60}, are currently manufactured by BARRX Medical, Inc., (Sunnyvale, CA, USA). Each device consists of tightly spaced electrodes (250 μm intervals) that deliver high-frequency radio waves, generating heat. The established energy density and dosimetry have been shown to cause a reliable depth of tissue injury to the level of the *muscularis mucosae*, deep enough to destroy the target epithelium, but not so deep as to injure the submucosa and cause subsequent stricture formation.

The balloon-based HALO^{360} is typically used for ablation of circumferential BE (Fig. 6.5). The ablation catheters, consisting of 3 cm of circumferential electrodes wrapped over a 4 cm balloon, come in a variety of diameters (18, 22, 25, 28 and 31 mm). A sizing balloon is initially utilized to select an ablation catheter of an appropriate diameter (Fig. 6.6). The ablation catheter is then advanced over a guidewire and positioned under endoscopic control at the upper limit of the target epithelium. Ablation is performed at an energy of 10 J/cm^2 (300 W/cm^2) for non-dysplastic BE and 12 J/cm^2 for LGD/HGD. If the length of BE is greater than 3 cm, the ablation catheter is advanced, positioned to have slight overlap with the initial segment, and ablation is repeated. Once all targeted areas have been treated, the ablation catheter is withdrawn and the coagulum is debrided from the esophageal mucosa. A specially designed cap that fits on the tip of the endoscope is available to facilitate this process. The ablation catheter is similarly cleaned then re-inserted. Ablation is repeated at each level such that two ablations are achieved across the entire segment of BE.

For smaller tongues or islands of BE, the HALO^{90} or HALO^{60} may be utilized (Fig. 6.7). The HALO^{90} is 13 mm wide and 20 mm in

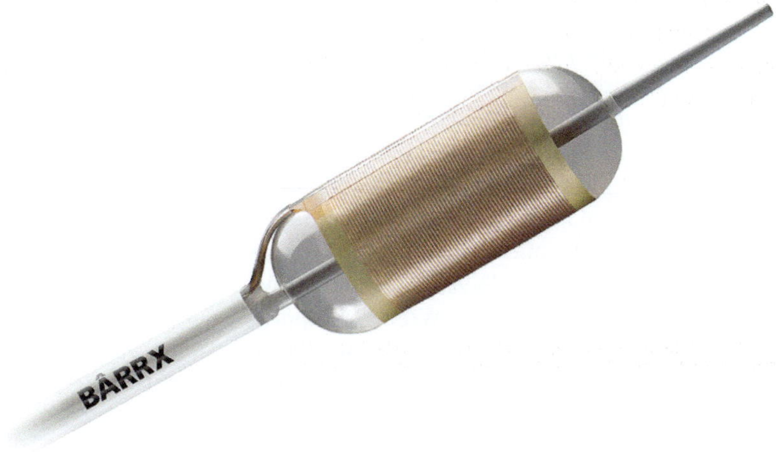

Fig. 6.5 HALO^{360} ablation catheter

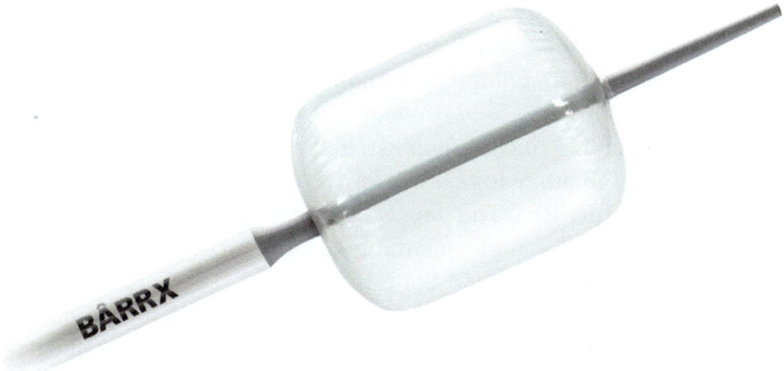

Fig. 6.6 Sizing balloon for the HALO^{360} ablation catheter

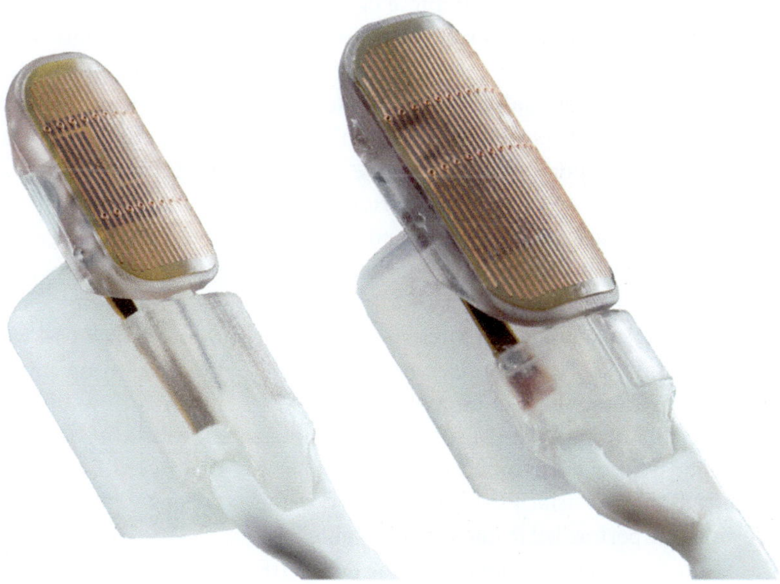

Fig. 6.7 HALO^{60} (*left*) and HALO^{90} (*right*)

length; the HALO[60] is slightly smaller. Each device is designed to fit over the tip of a standard adult flexible upper endoscope. The endoscope with attached device is inserted transorally, the target epithelium is ablated under direct endoscopic visualization, and ablation is repeated. The ablation catheter is repositioned to the next target zone, and the process carried out until all regions have been ablated. An energy level of 12 J/cm^2 (40 W/cm^2) is appropriate for both non-dysplastic and dysplastic BE. The coagulum is debrided using the tip of the device, the scope withdrawn, the ablation catheter cleaned, and the process is repeated. Thus, a total of four ablations are performed for each zone. Patients typically are brought back at 2-month intervals for repeat endoscopy and ablation until a complete response has been achieved.

Multiple studies have demonstrated the efficacy of RF ablation for both non-dysplastic and dysplastic BE. The most significant study to date was a multi-institutional trial from 20 centers in the United States, in which 127 patients with BE and low-grade dysplasia (LGD) or HGD were randomly assigned in a 2:1 fashion to RF ablation or sham treatment [23]. At a median follow-up of 12 months, 81 % of patients achieved complete eradication of HGD, 91 % complete eradication of LGD, and 77 % complete eradication of metaplasia on intention-to-treat analysis. The incidence of complications and side effects was quite low, with one case of hemorrhage and five patients (6 %) developing an esophageal stricture after ablation. Similar data have emerged for cryotherapy, though the technique has not been as extensively studied [24].

The experience with circumferential EMR for excising entire short or long segments of BE is emerging. While complete circumferential excision is feasible, a high rate of subsequent esophageal stenosis has been found (up to 88 % in a recent multicenter trial [25]), particularly if the excisions are performed in one session (Table 6.2). Based on these reports, ablation of residual BE appears preferable to stepwise circumferential resection.

Table 6.2 Results of step-wise radical resection of Barrett's esophagus compared to endoscopic resection of discrete nodules with ablation of non-nodular metaplasia

	SRER (*n* = 25)	ER/RFA (*n* = 22)
CR-Neoplasia	25 (100 %)	21 (96 %)
CR-IM	23 (92 %)	21 (96 %)
Metachronous neoplasia	1 (4 %)	0
Stenosis	88 %*	14 %*

From [25]

CR complete response rate, *IM* intestinal metaplasia, *SRER* stepwise radical endoscopic resection, *ER* endoscopic resection, *RFA* radiofrequency ablation

*$P < 0.001$

6.4 Comparative Studies Between Esophagectomy and Endoscopic Therapies for Early Esophageal Neoplasia

Three retrospective analyses have compared surgical and endoscopic treatment of BE with HGD or esophageal IMC. The first report, published in 2009, detailed the experience at the Mayo Clinic between 1998 and 2007. The series included 132 patients (74 %) treated endoscopically and 46 (26 %) treated via surgery [26]. The mean follow-up in the endoscopic cohort was 43 months. Seventy-five patients (57 %) underwent EMR alone, while 57 (43 %) were treated with a combination of EMR and PDT. The overall mortality was 17 %, and the metachronous cancer rate was 12 %. Of the 24 patients with persistent or recurrent cancer, 9 required esophagectomy, 1 underwent chemoradiation, and 14 were treated with repeat EMR. For the group undergoing esophagectomy, the mean follow-up was 64 months and the overall mortality was 20 %. The authors concluded that overall survival was comparable in the two groups.

The second report, published in 2011, described the experience at the University of

Table 6.3 Esophagectomy versus endoscopic resection for esophageal mucosal adenocarcinoma

	Complete response (%)	Major complications (%)	90-day mortality (%)	Recurrence rate (%)
Surgery	100	32	2.6	0
ER	98.7[a]	0	0	6.6[b]

From [28]
ER endoscopic resection
[a]Single patient died of other causes prior to complete response
[b]Repeat endoscopic therapy possible in all patients

Southern California in 101 patients with either HGD or IMC, 61 treated with esophagectomy and 40 via endoscopy [27]. No perioperative mortality occurred. The cohort treated endoscopically underwent a total of 109 EMRs and 70 ablation sessions. The median number of endoscopic interventions per patient was three. The metachronous neoplasia rate was 20 %, with three patients (7.5 %) requiring esophagectomy for endoscopic treatment failure. Comparing endoscopic and surgical therapy, the former was associated with lower morbidity (0 versus 39 %), though similar overall (94 % in both groups) and disease-free survival at 3 years.

The third report, also from 2011, compared outcomes between endoscopic and surgical therapy at two high-volume specialty centers in Germany [28]. Between 1996 and 2009, 38 patients underwent transthoracic esophagectomy with two-field lymphadenectomy for IMC at the University of Cologne. For comparison, 76 patients having undergone EMR and APC in Wiesbaden were matched for age, gender, depth of invasion, and differentiation. Similar to the other reports, endoscopic treatment was associated with equivalent neoplasia response rates, but with lower morbidity compared to esophagectomy and no mortality (Table 6.3).

Conclusions

Advances in endoscopic therapies have brought about a recent revolution in the treatment of early esophageal neoplasia. In the span of just a few years, the role of esophagectomy for cure of BE with HGD or IMC has been largely supplanted by equally effective, yet less morbid, endoscopic alternatives in appropriately selected patients. Esophagectomy will continue to have a role for patients unwilling to stay the course of a prolonged endoscopic treatment regimen or in cases difficult to manage by endoscopic means, and offers definitive therapy in a single intervention. Surgeons should offer surgical options with low morbidity and mortality, and that provide a good long-term quality of life, in order for esophageal resection to remain competitive as a treatment alternative. Various modalities of both EMR and endoscopic ablation have proven to be valuable tools in the armamentarium of physicians treating esophageal neoplasia and metaplasia. As with all new procedures, the esophagologist must possess an adequate understanding of the indications, strengths, limitations and potential pitfalls of the techniques in order to apply them in appropriately selected circumstances. A course of endoscopic therapy, while preferable in many cases, typically requires multiple sessions to achieve a complete response [29]. The patient must accept this fact in advance and be ready to commit to a prolonged period of treatment and surveillance. Compliance with the therapeutic regimen is critical; a challenge for the treating physician, therefore, is establishing and maintaining a system of follow-up over the course of years. Esophageal surgeons are well advised to incorporate the various endoscopic techniques into their therapeutic toolbox, as they have emerged as a new standard of care for BE with HGD or IMC.

Key Points

- Esophagectomy has been the standard of care for treatment of Barrett's esophagus with high-grade dysplasia or mucosal adenocarcinoma. In experienced hands, and with appropriately selected patients, esophagectomy in this setting is associated with an approximately 1 % perioperative mortality and reasonable morbidity, though with the potential to negatively impact gastrointestinal function
- When considering esophageal resection as an option for early esophageal neoplasia, the surgeon should choose an operation that avoids a thoracotomy and offers both low perioperative morbidity as well as good long-term quality of life. Options include a transhiatal esophagectomy, with or without sparing of the vagus nerves, and minimally invasive esophagectomy
- Endoscopic therapies, including techniques for endoscopic resection and ablation, have emerged as a new standard of care for the majority of cases of early esophageal neoplasia. Cure rates following endoscopic treatment paradigms in appropriately selected patients rival those achieved by esophagectomy, but with lower short and long-term morbidity
- Endoscopic resection should be performed on discrete mucosal nodules in the setting of Barrett's esophagus, both to facilitate accurate diagnosis and staging as well as to cure small foci of neoplasia limited to the mucosa. The remaining non-nodular Barrett's esophagus should subsequently be ablated to eliminate occult synchronous or metachronous neoplasia
- A course of endoscopic treatment for early esophageal neoplasia may require multiple sessions and requires compliance by both the patient and the treating physician

References

1. Spechler SJ, Sharma P, Souza RF et al (2011) American Gastroenterological Association medical position statement on the management of Barrett's esophagus. Gastroenterology 140:1084–1091
2. Williams VA, Watson TJ, Herbella FA et al (2007) Esophagectomy for high grade dysplasia is safe, curative and results in good alimentary outcome. J Gastrointest Surg 11:1589–1597
3. Schnell TG, Sontag SJ, Chejfec G et al (2001) Long-term nonsurgical management of Barrett's esophagus with high-grade dysplasia. Gastroenterology 120: 1607–1619
4. Barr H (2003) Ablative mucosectomy is the procedure of choice to prevent Barrett's cancer. Gut 52(1):14–15
5. Bailey SH, Bull DA, Harpole DH et al (2003) Outcomes after esophagectomy: a ten-year prospective cohort. Ann Thorac Surg 75:217–222
6. Connors RC, Reuben BC, Neumayer LA, Bull DA (2007) Comparing outcomes after transthoracic and transhiatal esophagectomy: a 5-year prospective cohort of 17,395 patients. J Am Coll Surg 205:735–740
7. Portale G, Hagen JA, Peters JH et al (2006) Modern 5-year survival of resectable esophageal adenocarcinoma: single institution experience with 263 patients. J Am Coll Surg 202:588–596
8. Orringer MB, Marshall B, Chang AC et al (2007) Two thousand transhiatal esophagectomies: changing trends, lessons learned. Ann Surg 246:363–374
9. Swanson SJ, Batirel HF, Bueno R et al (2001) Transthoracic esophagectomy with radical mediastinal and abdominal lymph node dissection and cervical esophagogastrostomy for esophageal carcinoma. Ann Thorac Surg 72:1918–1925
10. Hulscher JB, Tijssen JG, Obertop H, van Lanschot JJ (2001) Transthoracic versus transhiatal resection for carcinoma of the esophagus: a meta-analysis. Ann Thorac Surg 72:306–313
11. Fernando HC, Luketich JD, Buenaventura PO et al (2002) Outcomes of minimally invasive esophagectomy (MIE) for high-grade dysplasia of the esophagus. Eur J Cardiothorac Surg 22:1–6
12. Peyre CG, DeMeester SR, Rizzetto C et al (2007) Vagal-sparing esophagectomy: the ideal operation for intramucosal adenocarcinoma and Barrett's with high-grade dysplasia. Ann Surg 246:665–671
13. Inoue H, Endo M, Takeshita K et al (1992) A new simplified technique of endoscopic esophageal mucosal resection using a cap-fitted panendoscope. Surg Endosc 6:264–265
14. Rice TW, Zuccaro G Jr, Adelstein DJ et al (1998) Esophageal carcinoma: depth of tumor invasion is predictive of regional nodal status. Ann Thorac Surg 65:787–792

15. Buskens CJ, Westerterp M, Lagarde SM et al (2004) Prediction of appropriateness of local endoscopic treatment for high-grade dysplasia and early adenocarcinomas by EUS and histopathologic features. Gastrointest Endosc 60:703–707
16. Liu L, Hofstetter WL, Rashid A et al (2005) Significance of the depth of tumor invasion and lymph node metastasis in superficially invasive (T1) esophageal adenocarcinoma. Am J Surg Pathol 29:1079–1085
17. Altorki NK, Lee PC, Liss Y et al (2008) Multifocal neoplasia and nodal metastases in T1 esophageal carcinoma: implications for endoscopic treatment. Ann Surg 247:434–439
18. Sepesi B, Watson TJ, Zhou D et al (2010) Are endoscopic therapies appropriate for superficial submucosal esophageal adenocarcinoma? An analysis of esophagectomy specimens. J Am Coll Surg 210:418–427
19. Leers JM, DeMeester SR, Oezcelik A et al (2011) The prevalence of lymph node metastases in patients with T1 esophageal adenocarcinoma: a retrospective review of esophagectomy specimens. Ann Surg 253:271–278
20. May A, Gossner L, Behrens A et al (2003) A prospective randomized trial of two different endoscopic resection techniques in 100 consecutive resections in patients with early cancer of the esophagus. Gastrointest Endosc 58:167–175
21. Ell C, May A, Pech O et al (2007) Curative endoscopic resection of early esophageal adenocarcinomas (Barrett's cancer). Gastrointest Endosc 65:3–10
22. Pech O, Behrens A, May A et al (2008) Long-term results and risk factor analysis for recurrence after curative endoscopic therapy in 349 patients with high-grade intraepithelial neoplasia and mucosal adenocarcinoma in Barrett's oesophagus. Gut 57:1200–1206
23. Shaheen NJ, Sharma P, Overholt BF et al (2009) Radiofrequency ablation in Barrett's esophagus with dysplasia. N Eng J Med 360:2277–2288
24. Greenwald BD, Dumot JA, Horwhat JD, Lightdale CJ, Abrams JA (2010) Safety, tolerability, and efficacy of endoscopic low-pressure liquid nitrogen spray cryotherapy in the esophagus. Dis Esophagus 23:13–19
25. van Vilsteren FGI, Pouw RE, Seewald S et al (2011) Stepwise radical endoscopic resection versus radiofrequency ablation for Barrett's oesophagus with high-grade dysplasia or early cancer: a multicentre randomised trial. Gut 60(6):765–773
26. Prasad GA, Wu TT, Wigle DA et al (2009) Endoscopic and surgical treatment of mucosal (T1a) esophageal adenocarcinoma in Barrett's esophagus. Gastroenterology 137:816–823
27. Zehetner J, DeMeester SR, Hagen JA et al (2011) Endoscopic resection and ablation versus esophagectomy for high-grade dysplasia and intramucosal adenocarcinoma. J Thorac Cardiovasc Surg 141:39–47
28. Pech O, Bollschweiler E, Manner H et al (2011) Comparison between endoscopic and surgical resection of mucosal adenocarcinoma in Barrett's esophagus at two high-volume centers. Ann Surg 254:67–72
29. Galey KM, Wilshire CL, Watson TJ et al (2011) Endoscopic management of early esophageal neoplasia: an emerging standard. J Gastrointest Surg 15: 1299–1302

7 Cost-Effectiveness of Radiofrequency Ablation for Barrett's Esophagus

Francesca Rancati and Emanuele Meroni

Based on over 70 peer-reviewed publications and experience from more than 100,000 radiofrequency ablation (RFA) procedures performed in some 46 countries worldwide, the HALO Ablation System represents a device that is changing the treatment paradigm for patients with Barrett's esophagus. RFA has demonstrated high rates of complete histological eradication of intestinal metaplasia and dysplasia with an exceptional safety profile [1, 2]. Durability of the effect and a reduction in cancer progression have been demonstrated [3]. RFA has also proven to be more cost-effective than endoscopic surveillance in all grades of Barrett's esophagus [4, 5] and to yield a better quality of life at less cost than esophagectomy or other ablative strategies in high grade dysplasia patients [6, 7].

Historically, early Barrett's esophagus, low grade dysplasia (LGD) and non-dysplastic Barrett's esophagus (NDBE) have simply been endoscopically surveyed. However, as stated in the 2011 American Gastroenterological Association (AGA) guidelines, "endoscopic surveillance has never been proven to prevent or reduce deaths from esophageal cancer" [8]. No randomized controlled trials exist to support its clinical efficacy in Barrett's esophagus.

One of the biggest issues surrounding surveillance is its inability to detect step-wise progression of Barrett's from NDBE to invasive cancer. Sharma et al. reported that over 50 % of patients who developed high grade dysplasia (HGD) or cancer while undergoing surveillance did not have prior findings of dysplasia [9]. In addition, even with the availability of high resolution endoscopy and chromoendoscopy, i.e. narrow band imaging (NBI), sampling error is a major shortcoming of surveillance programs. The observers' intervariability is high, even among expert gastrointestinal pathologists. Patients are uncomfortable about having a pre-cancerous condition simply watched. Last but not least, surveillance has never been found to be cost-effective.

On the contrary, cost-utility studies have been conducted in the United States and Europe to prove the effectiveness of RFA treatment in Barrett's esophagus.

Inadomi et al. compared the cost-benefit of surveillance versus ablation versus esophagectomy in patients at all grades of Barrett's esophagus: intestinal metaplasia (IM), LGD and HGD [4].

F. Rancati
Medical Affairs Department, Bârrx Medical, Inc,
Via Novara 30, Malnate (VA), Italy
e-mail: francesca.rancati@covidien.com

E. Meroni (✉)
Department of Diagnostic Endoscopy
and Endoscopic Surgery,
Istituto Nazionale Tumori, Via Venezian 1, Milan, Italy
e-mail: emanuele.meroni@istitutotumori.mi.it

L. Bonavina (ed.), *Innovation in Esophageal Surgery*,
DOI 10.1007/978-88-470-2469-4_7, © Springer-Verlag Italia 2012

A decision analysis model was created to examine a population of patients with Barrett's esophagus (mean age 50 years), with separate analyses for patients with and without dysplasia. Strategies compared were: no endoscopic surveillance; endoscopic surveillance with ablation for incident dysplasia; immediate ablation followed by endoscopic surveillance in all patients or limited to patients in whom metaplasia persisted; and esophagectomy. Ablation modalities modeled included radiofrequency, argon plasma coagulation, multipolar electrocoagulation and photodynamic therapy. Endoscopic ablation for patients with HGD was found to increase life expectancy by 3 quality-adjusted years at an incremental cost compared with no intervention. Patients with LGD or no dysplasia could also be optimally managed with ablation, but continued surveillance after eradication of metaplasia was expensive. If ablation could permanently eradicate at least 28 % of LGD or 40 % of non-dysplastic metaplasias, ablation would be preferred to surveillance.

Das et al. [5] evaluated, using a Markov model, three competing strategies for a hypothetical 50-year-old cohort with NDBE: natural history, surveillance and RFA. Strategy I – natural history of Barrett's disease (without surveillance); Strategy II – surveillance performed according to the American College of Gastroenterology practice guidelines [10]; Strategy III – endoscopic ablative therapy. The model was biased against ablative therapy with a conservative estimate of complete response and continued standard surveillance even after complete ablation. All potential complications were accounted for, and an incomplete histological response after ablation was presumed to have the same risk of progression as untreated Barrett's. Transitional probabilities, discounted cost, and utility values to estimate quality-adjusted life-years (QALYs) were obtained from published information. Direct costs were used in the analysis.

In the baseline analysis, the ablative strategy yielded the highest QALY and was more cost-effective than endoscopic surveillance. In a Monte Carlo analysis, the relative risk of developing cancer in the strategy based on endoscopic ablation was decreased compared with the other strategies. In threshold analysis, the critical determinants of cost-effectiveness of the ablative strategy were rate of complete response to ablation, total cost of ablation, and risk of progression to dysplasia.

The authors determined that RFA is the most cost-effective strategy and results in the highest QALYs and lowest risk for cancer, within the limits of the model. Their conclusion was that "ablation for NDBE is more cost-effective than surveillance".

In Europe, the cost effectiveness of endoscopic therapy, including RFA, has been compared to esophagectomy in high grade dysplasia/early esophageal adenocarcinoma patients. Surgical therapy is indeed associated with increased operative mortality and morbidity, but possibly a decreased recurrence rate compared with endoscopic therapy when using endoscopic mucosal resection (EMR) and radiofrequency ablation.

Pohl et al. [6] compared the cost-effectiveness of esophagectomy and endoscopic therapy in the treatment of early esophageal adenocarcinoma. A decision analysis model was made, using the incremental cost- effectiveness ratio as the main outcome measurement.

During the 5-year study period, endoscopic therapy cost $17,000.00 and yielded 4.88 QALYs, compared with $28,000.00 and 4.59, respectively, for esophagectomy. Varying the recurrence rates of cancer or Barrett's esophagus metaplasia after endoscopic therapy did not change the overall outcome. The sensitivity analysis demonstrated, however, that the outcome depended on the rate of lymph node involvement and operative mortality. Under the best of circumstances in favor of esophagectomy – such as 2 % operative mortality, no reduced quality of life after esophagectomy, and a low 5-year survival rate after recurrence of endoscopic ablation – the risk of positive lymph nodes still needed to exceed 25 % before esophagectomy became the preferred treatment option. This threshold is twice as high as the values reported for early submucosal cancer invasion.

Even though the data available on the long-term outcome of EMR and RFA are limited, it was found that endoscopic therapy for early Barrett's esophagus adenocarcinoma is more effective and less expensive than esophagectomy. Even in early esophageal adenocarcinoma with submucosal invasion, endoscopic therapy is a cost-effective alternative to esophagectomy, especially in patients with a high operative risk.

Boger et al. [7] compared the cost-benefit of esophagectomy versus RFA for patients with high-grade dysplasia. They constructed a Markov model to simulate the natural history of a cohort of patients with HGD in Barrett's esophagus undergoing one of two treatment options: esophagectomy or RFA followed by endoscopic surveillance with esophagectomy for HGD recurrence or persistence.

In the base case analysis, radiofrequency ablation dominated as it generated 0.4 extra QALYs at a cost savings of £1,902.00. For esophagectomy to be the most cost-effective option, it required a radiofrequency ablation treatment failure rate (HGD persistence or progression to cancer) of >44 %, or an annual risk of HGD recurrence or progression to cancer in the ablated esophagus of >15 % per annum. There was an 85 % probability that RFA remained cost-effective at the NICE willingness to pay threshold range of £20,000–30,000. The authors stated that RFA is likely to be a cost-effective option for HGD in Barrett's esophagus in the UK, "yielding more quality of life at less cost than surveillance, esophagectomy or other ablative strategies…".

In conclusion, RFA is a promising treatment in Barrett's esophagus in terms of cost-effectiveness in comparison to other treatments. As further post-ablation data become available, the optimal management strategy will be clarified. There are still unclear issues that require to be investigated, especially to establish RFA effectiveness in the long term and to decide which patients without dysplasia are at risk of malignant progression and would benefit from the ablative treatment.

Key Points

- Endoscopic ablation by radiofrequency is changing the treatment paradigm for patients with Barrett's esophagus
- The procedure appears safe, effective, and durable
- It has also proven to be more cost-effective than endoscopic surveillance in all grades of Barrett's esophagus and to yield a better quality of life at less cost than esophagectomy or other ablative strategies in high grade dysplasia patients

References

1. Shaheen NJ, Sharma P, Overholt BF et al (2009) Radiofrequency ablation in Barrett's esophagus with dysplasia. N Engl J Med 360(22):2277–2288
2. Fleischer DE, Overholt BF, Sharma VK et al (2010) Endoscopic radiofrequency ablation for Barrett's esophagus: 5-year outcomes from a prospective multicenter trial. Endoscopy 42:781–789
3. Shaheen NJ et al (2011) Durability of radiofrequency ablation in Barrett's esophagus with dysplasia. Gastroenterology 141:460–468
4. Inadomi JM, Somsouk M, Madanick RD, Thomas JP, Shaheen NJ (2009) A cost-utility analysis of ablative therapy for Barrett's esophagus. Gastroenterology 136:2101–2114
5. Das A, Wells C, Kim HJ, Fleischer DE, Crowell MD, Sharma VK (2009) An economic analysis of endoscopic ablative therapy for management of nondysplastic Barrett's esophagus. Endoscopy 41:400–408
6. Pohl H, Sonnenberg A, Strobel S, Eckardt A, Roesch T (2009) Endoscopic versus surgical therapy for early cancer in Barrett's esophagus: a decision analysis. Gastrointest Endosc 70:623–631
7. Boger PC, Turner D, Roderick P, Patel P (2010) A UK-based cost-utility analysis of radiofrequency ablation or oesophagectomy for the management of high-grade dysplasia in Barrett's esophagus. Aliment Pharmacol Ther 32:1332–1342
8. American Gastroenterological Association (2011) Medical position statement on the management of Barrett's esophagus. Gastroenterology 140:1084–1091
9. Sharma P, Falk GW, Weston AP et al (2006) Dysplasia and cancer in a large multicenter cohort of patients with Barrett's esophagus. Clin Gastroenterol Hepatol 4:566–572
10. Wang C, Sampliner RE (2008) Updated guidelines 2008 for the diagnosis, surveillance, and therapy of Barrett's esophagus. Am J Gastroenterol 97:1888–1895

Vagal-Sparing Esophagectomy

8

Steven R. DeMeester

8.1 Scope of the Problem

Once a rare tumor, adenocarcinoma of the esophagus is currently the cancer with the fastest rising incidence in America. Recent data indicate that in the US since 1975 the rate of increase of adenocarcinoma of the esophagus has outpaced the next closest cancer, melanoma, by nearly three times [1–3]. In addition to the increasing prevalence of the disease, surveillance programs for patients with Barrett's esophagus have led to the identification of increasing numbers of patients with high-grade dysplasia or early-stage esophageal adenocarcinomas. Although esophagectomy is curative in the majority of these patients, associated morbidity and mortality remain a hurdle for patient acceptance of the procedure.

In an effort to minimize the morbidity associated with an esophagectomy surgeons have developed minimally invasive techniques as well as methods to spare the vagus nerves and thereby reduce the incidence of post-vagotomy diarrhea and dumping symptoms. The combination of these concepts, a laparoscopic vagal-sparing esophagectomy, is perhaps the optimal procedure to minimize the early and long-term morbidity of an esophagectomy while still providing curative therapy for patients with high-grade dysplasia or intramucosal adenocarcinoma. However, the vagal-sparing procedure does not remove lymph nodes, and it is therefore not appropriate for tumors that penetrate into the submucosa and have a significant risk of lymph node metastases. Consequently, it is critical to determine the depth of invasion of any visible lesion within the Barrett's mucosa prior to consideration of a vagal-sparing approach. Endoscopic ultrasound is not accurate enough to determine the "T" stage of these superficial lesions [4–7]. Therefore any visible lesion should be excised using endoscopic resection, and the depth of invasion pathologically determined [8].

8.2 Technique of Vagal-Sparing Esophagectomy

The vagal-sparing esophagectomy was originally described by Akiyama [9]. We adopted this technique and to date more than 150 patients with high-grade dysplasia and/or intramucosal cancer, or benign conditions including end-stage achalasia and reflux disease, have undergone an open or laparoscopic vagal-sparing procedure. The stomach was the preferred esophageal substitute in most patients, although a colon interposition was performed in some. Vagal integrity was tested in a subgroup of patients using sham feeding, pancreatic polypeptide measurements, Congo-red staining, and scintigraphic gastric emptying

S.R. DeMeester
Department of Surgery, Keck School of Medicine, University of Southern California, 1510 San Pablo St, Suite 514, Los Angeles, CA 90033, USA
e-mail: sdemeester@surgery.usc.edu

L. Bonavina (ed.), *Innovation in Esophageal Surgery*,
DOI 10.1007/978-88-470-2469-4_8,

studies. The follow-up evaluation of these patients demonstrated that this nerve-sparing operation is associated with a significant decrease in the prevalence of dumping and diarrhea compared to patients who underwent a standard esophagectomy with vagotomy [10].

Vagal-sparing procedures are performed in a similar way to a transhiatal operation except that the esophagus is stripped from the mediastinum and no mediastinal or transhiatal dissection is done. The procedure starts in the abdomen; the hiatus is opened and both vagal trunks are encircled with a vessel-loop. The nerves are gently retracted toward the patient's right, and the gastroesophageal fat pad is dissected beginning on the left of the esophagogastric junction to allow the anterior vagus nerve to be brought to the right of the esophagus. This is done to avoid inadvertent injury of the anterior vagus nerve. A highly selective vagotomy is then performed starting just above the crow's foot. This step is necessary if the stomach will be used as the esophageal substitute, and is beneficial in case of colon interposition to reduce gastric secretion and the incidence of graft ulceration. The highly selective vagotomy is facilitated by sequential grasping of the lesser curve with Babcock clamps and by using the harmonic scalpel to prevent bleeding that may cause inadvertent injury to the distal vagal branches. Upon completion of the vagotomy, the gastroesophageal junction should be completely exposed and the lesser curve above the crow's foot skeletonized. The greater curve is mobilized in the same fashion as for a standard gastric pull-up when the stomach has been chosen as the esophageal substitute. Conversely, when the colon has been chosen as replacement, the greater omentum is detached from the transverse colon and a tunnel from the lesser sac to the hiatus for the colon graft is created by dividing the most proximal short gastric and the posterior pancreatico-gastric vessels. The colon is usually mobilized based on the ascending branch of the left colic artery. The distance from the tip of the left ear to the xiphoid is measured with an umbilical tape, and required length of colon is marked out by measuring a similar distance starting from the point where the left colic vessels tether the graft. The colon can be safely divided at this point and placed in the pelvis for later use [11].

The esophagus is exposed through a left neck incision and encircled with a penrose drain. The upper mediastinal portion of the esophagus is then dissected bluntly with a finger. A nasogastric tube is temporarily inserted and used to irrigate the esophagus with a diluted iodine solution. Through a small gastrotomy near the gastroesophageal junction, a standard vein stripper is passed retrograde up the esophagus and brought out the anterior wall of the cervical esophagus. Alternatively, the cardia is divided with a stapler and a small portion of the staple line is opened to provide access to the esophageal lumen. The cervical esophagus is divided at the site where the vein stripper comes out. The divided distal end of the esophagus is then suture ligated and tied securely using endo-loops to prevent slippage and incomplete stripping of the esophagus. By pulling the vein stripper from below, the esophagus is inverted on itself. A long umbilical tape is tied to the distal end of the cervical esophagus to provide access to the posterior mediastinal tract after the esophagus has been stripped. After the stripping maneuver, the esophagus appears inverted with the mucosa external to the muscular wall. In general, very little force is required to pull the esophagus out and bleeding is minimal. Excessive resistance should raise concern and should prompt conversion to a transhiatal procedure.

In patients with Barrett's esophagus and high-grade dysplasia or intramucosal cancer, all layers of the esophagus are stripped out so as not to inadvertently leave any Barrett's tissue or tumor behind. Conversely, in patients with benign conditions such as achalasia only the esophageal mucosa need be stripped out. In such circumstances, a cervical esophageal myotomy is made. The mucosa is encircled with a ligature, secured with a tie and stripped from below, leaving the remaining muscular wall of the esophagus in place.

After the esophagus has been removed, dilatation of the mediastinal tract is necessary to prevent constriction of the graft. We use a 90 cc balloon Foley catheter progressively filled with

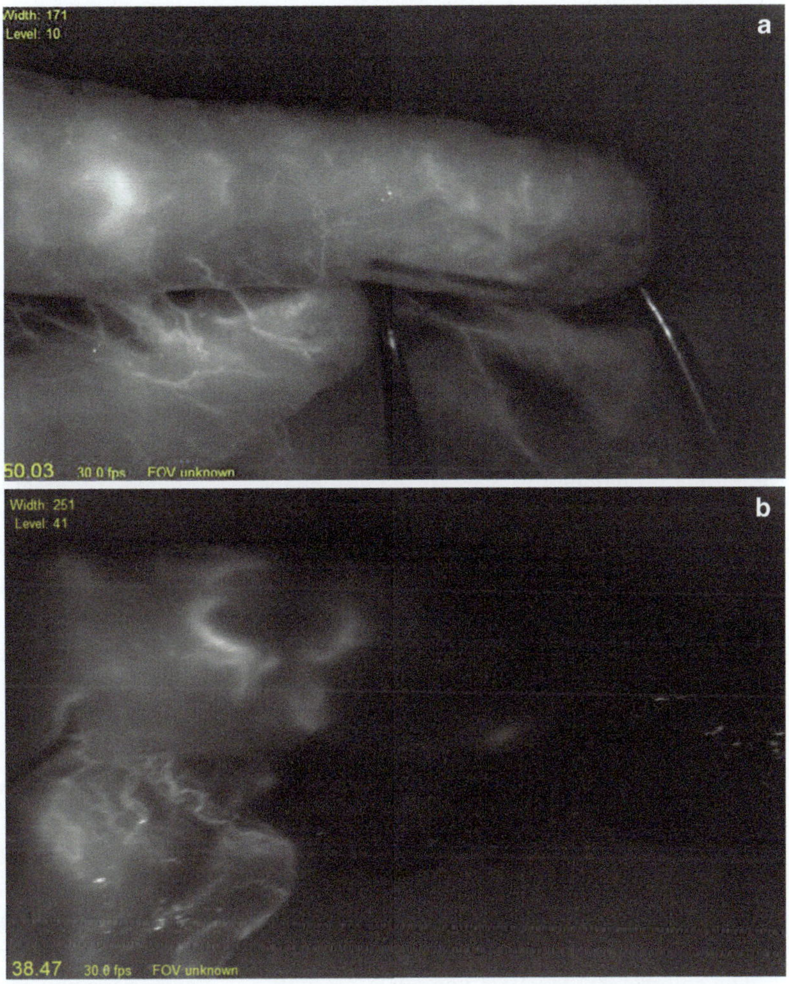

Fig. 8.1 (**a**) SPY image showing well perfused graft in which any point can be chosen for the anastomosis. (**b**) SPY image showing line of demarcation from good (*left*) to compromised (*right*) perfusion. Anastomosis is done to the well-perfused area

saline and pulled up through the mediastinum two or three times to ensure that an adequate tunnel is created. This is particularly important in patients with a normal caliber esophagus. The graft can then be brought up through the posterior mediastinal tract.

In patients undergoing a gastric pull-up, the stomach tube is fashioned leaving the crow's foot intact and no pyloroplasty is performed since the antral innervation has been spared. The vascular supply of the gastric tube is typically excellent since the left gastric artery has been preserved and only the branches to the skeletonized lesser curve region were divided. We confirm the perfusion of the graft using SPY technology, and in this way ensure the anastomosis is done to a well-perfused area of the graft (Fig. 8.1). At this point, the gastric tube is pulled up through the posterior mediastinum and a cervical esophago-gastric anastomosis is constructed in a standard fashion. After completing the anastomosis, the graft is gently pulled back into the abdomen to eliminate redundancy and is sutured to the crura to prevent transhiatal herniation of abdominal contents.

In patients undergoing colon interposition, the whole innervated stomach is left intact and only the cardia is excised. A highly selective vagotomy is performed along the lesser curvature to reduce acid secretion and prevent the development of colo-gastric anastomotic ulcers. An extensive mobilization of the greater curvature is not required. Instead, only the most proximal short gastric vessels along with the posterior pancreatico-duodenal vessels are divided in order to create a window near the left crus of the diaphragm. The colon graft is tunnellized up *posterior* to the stomach through this window, into the hiatus, and then up through the posterior mediastinum. In patients with achalasia, in whom only the mucosa was stripped out through an anterior gastrotomy, the whole muscular tube of the native esophagus remains intact; therefore, a sufficient sized hole must be cut into the tube on the left side near the hiatus to allow the colon graft to be pulled up inside the residual muscular tube. In patients with high-grade dysplasia or intramucosal adenocarcinoma, in whom all layers of the esophagus have been stripped out, this issue does not exist since only the mediastinal tract is present at the hiatus. The esophago-colonic anastomosis can be performed either with a stapled or hand-sewn technique. If the muscular tube of the esophagus has been preserved it can be pulled up to cover the anastomosis like a sheath. The colon is then gently pulled back into the abdomen to avoid redundancy and sutured to the left crus of the diaphragm to prevent graft twisting or transhiatal herniation of abdominal contents. Sutures should be placed between the colon graft and the posterior aspect of the hiatus near the crura decussation since a hernia can occur underneath the colon graft.

The colon is divided 10–15 cm distal from the hiatus and attention should be paid not to injure the vascular arcade. A stapled colo-gastric anastomosis is done to the posterior wall of the proximal fundus using a 75 mm gastrointestinal anastomosis (GIA) stapler. Finally, the colocolostomy is accomplished in a standard fashion taking care to avoid traction on the left colic vessels and the marginal artery supplying the graft. Typically this requires that the right colon be brought up into the left upper quadrant.

The vagal-sparing procedure is readily adapted to a fully laparoscopic approach if a gastric pull-up is planned. The gastric mobilization as well as the highly selective vagotomy are straightforward laparoscopic procedures. Placement of a hand-port through a 4 cm midline incision facilitates stripping of the esophagus, subsequent dilatation of the mediastinal tract, and pull-up of the graft attached to a chest tube. Similar to an open procedure, the gastric tube should be sutured to the left crus to prevent twisting of the graft or mediastinal herniation of abdominal contents.

Conclusions

An increasing number of patients with high-grade dysplasia or early-stage Barrett adenocarcinoma are being identified through surveillance programs and a more liberal use of upper gastrointestinal endoscopy. The length of the Barrett's segment, the presence of a ulcer or nodule within the Barrett's segment, and the age and overall patient fitness influence the choice of treatment. Endoscopic mucosal resection should represent the first-line approach in these patients because of the potential to reliably determine the depth of invasion of superficial cancers. This has a significant impact on therapeutic strategy since submucosal invasion carries a high risk of lymph node metastases and therapies that do not include a lymphadenectomy are potentially inadequate. A vagal-sparing esophagectomy has the advantage to eliminate all Barrett's tissue while minimizing the morbidity resulting from the traditional techniques of esophagectomy that include a vagotomy. The applicability of this operation to a laparoscopic approach should encourage physician and patient acceptance.

Key Points

- Identification of high-grade dysplasia or early stage adenocarcinoma is increasing
- Associated morbidity and mortality remain a hurdle for patient acceptance of esophagectomy
- Vagal-sparing esophagectomy minimizes the morbidity of an esophagectomy, particularly the dumping and diarrhea associated with vagotomy
- Submucosal invasion imparts a significant risk of lymph node metastases and therapies that do not include a lymphadenectomy are potentially inadequate

References

1. Blot WJ, Devesa SS, Kneller RW, Fraumeni JFJ (1991) Rising incidence of adenocarcinoma of the esophagus and gastric cardia [see comments]. JAMA 265:1287–1289
2. Kubo A, Corley DA (2004) Marked multi-ethnic variation of esophageal and gastric cardia carcinomas within the United States. Am J Gastroenterol 99:582–588
3. Pohl H, Welch HG (2005) The role of overdiagnosis and reclassification in the marked increase of esophageal adenocarcinoma incidence. J Natl Cancer Inst 97:142–146
4. Buttar N, Nijhawan P, Krishnadath K et al (2000) Combined endoscopic mucosal resection (EMR) and photodynamic therapy (PDT) for esophageal neoplasia within Barrett's esophagus. Gastroenterology 118:A405
5. Heidemann J, Schilling MK, Schmassmann A et al (2000) Accuracy of endoscopic ultrasonography in preoperative staging of esophageal carcinoma. Dig Surg 17:219–224
6. Menzel J, Hoepffner N, Nottberg H et al (1999) Preoperative staging of esophageal carcinoma: miniprobe sonography versus conventional endoscopic ultrasound in a prospective histopathologically verified study [comment]. Endoscopy 31:291–297
7. Hunerbein M, Ulmer C, Handke T, Schlag PM (2003) Endosonography of upper gastrointestinal tract cancer on demand using miniprobes or endoscopic ultrasound. Surg Endosc 17:615–619
8. Maish MS, DeMeester SR (2004) Endoscopic mucosal resection as a staging technique to determine the depth of invasion of esophageal adenocarcinoma. Ann Thorac Surg 78:1777–1782
9. Akiyama H, Tsurumaru M, Kawamura T, Ono Y (1982) Esophageal stripping with preservation of the vagus nerve. Int Surg 67:125–128
10. Banki F, Mason RJ, DeMeester SR et al (2002) Vagal-sparing esophagectomy: a more physiologic alternative. Ann Surg 236:324–335; discussion 335–326
11. DeMeester SR (2001) Colon interposition following esophagectomy. Dis Esophagus 14:169–172

Thoracoscopic Esophagectomy

9

Miguel A. Cuesta, Donald L. van der Peet,
Surya S.A.Y. Biere, Suzanne S. Gisbertz,
and Mark van Berge Henegouwen

9.1 Introduction

The global incidence of esophageal cancer has increased by 30 % in the past two decades; in 1990, 316,000 people were diagnosed with esophageal cancer while in 2008, 482,300 new cases of esophageal cancer were recorded [1, 2]. Surgical resection with radical lymphadenectomy – usually after neoadjuvant chemotherapy or chemoradiotherapy – is considered the only curative option for resectable esophageal cancer [3–5].

Open esophagectomy performed through a right thoracotomy and laparotomy puts at least half the patients at risk for developing pulmonary complications. This necessitates prolonged stay in intensive care units and hospital wards and leads to consequences for the postoperative quality of life. Current mortality rates of esophageal resection are less than 5 % [6].

Minimally invasive esophagectomy (MIE), by avoiding thoracotomy and laparotomy, may reduce the rate of pulmonary infections, thereby resulting in a shorter hospital stay [7, 8]. Because of these potential advantages MIE is increasingly implemented in specialized centers.

M.A. Cuesta (✉) • D.L. van der Peet • S.S.A.Y. Biere • S.S. Gisbertz
Department of Surgery,
VU University Medical Centre,
Amsterdam, The Netherlands
e-mail: ma.cuesta@vumc.nl

M. van Berge Henegouwen
Department of Surgery,
Academic Medical Centre,
Amsterdam, The Netherlands

9.2 Advantages of Minimally Invasive Esophagectomy for Cancer

There is a general consensus in the literature that all esophageal cancers should be operated through the thorax and abdomen, i.e. two-field lymphadenectomy, in order to obtain an adequate radical resection with negative margins (longitudinal and radial), after a well tolerated neoadjuvant therapy (e.g. CROSS scheme). Only in patients with cardiac or respiratory comorbidity or elderly patients with tumors located very distally or at the gastroesophageal (GE) junction may a transhiatal approach be considered the approach of choice [9–18].

Why to perform the esophageal resection by MIE? What are the potential advantages of MIE? We hold these to be less trauma, no necessity for laparotomy and thoracotomy incisions, a better visualization of the operative field, no necessity of total pulmonary block, and less postoperative complications. Moreover, a transhiatal procedure performed laparoscopically allows a better view of the lower mediastinum, less displacement of the heart and a greater hemodynamic stability during operation [13]. The ultimate speculation is that a less traumatic operation will positively affect patient survival.

L. Bonavina (ed.), *Innovation in Esophageal Surgery*,
DOI 10.1007/978-88-470-2469-4_9, © Springer-Verlag Italia 2012

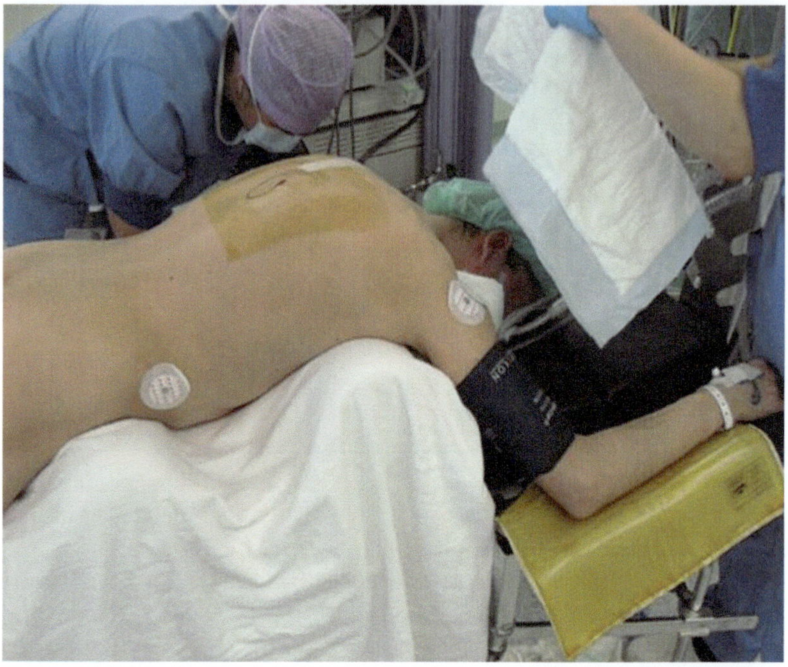

Fig. 9.1 The patient is positioned in the prone decubitus position

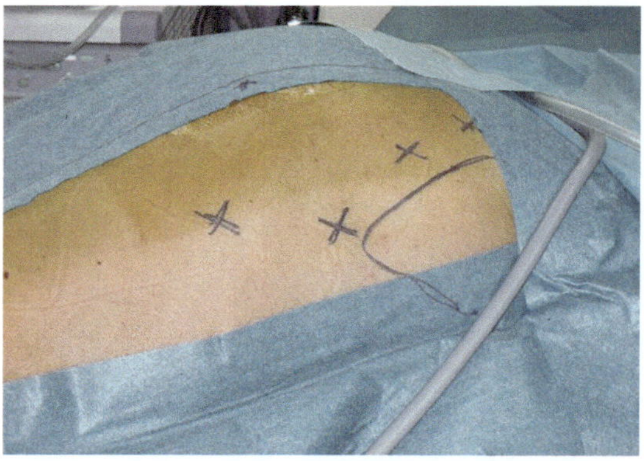

Fig. 9.2 Placement of trocars for the thoracoscopy

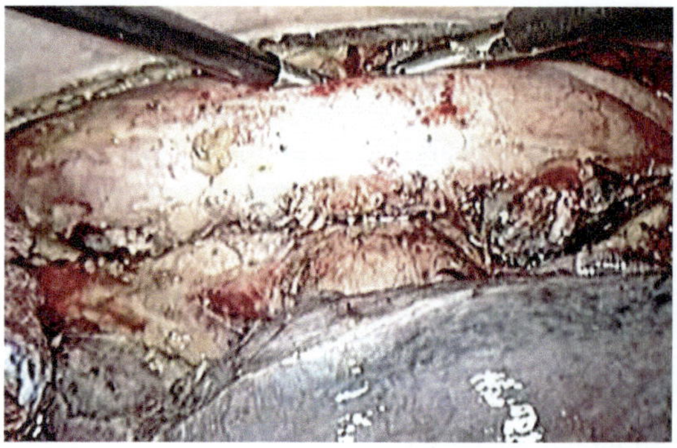

Fig. 9.3 Dissection of the esophagus with pleura

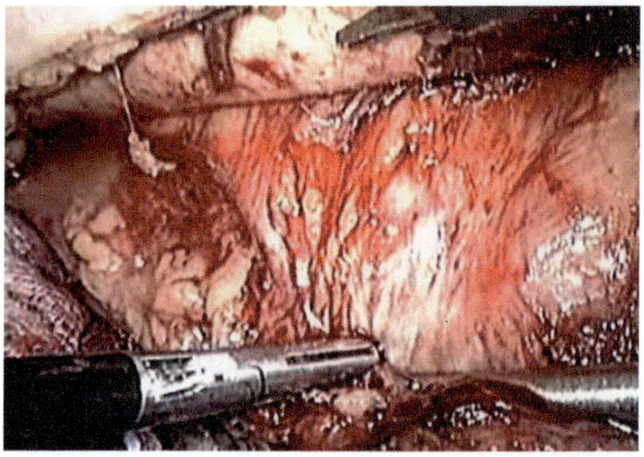

Fig. 9.4 The esophagus is dissected from the aorta and contralateral pleura

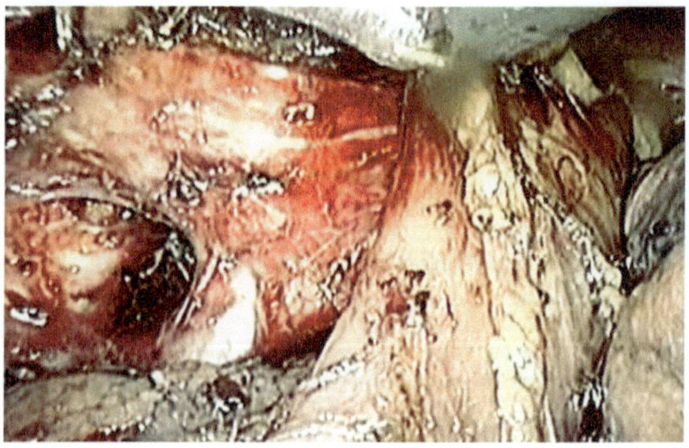

Fig. 9.5 Lymphadenectomy of the carina

Table 9.1 Possibilities of minimal access esophagectomy

Transhiatal esophagectomy	Da Palma, Bonavina, Cuesta
Right thoracoscopy + laparoscopy + cervical anastomosis	Dallemagne, Luketich
Ivor Lewis operation combined with laparoscopy	Luketich
Thoracoscopy in prone position	Cuschieri, Palanivelu, Cuesta
Robot assisted thoracoscopic combined with laparoscopy	van Hillegersberg Puntambekar

Table 9.1 shows all the conventional interventions by MIE. Thoracoscopic esophageal resection can be performed in the lateral position or in the prone position [7, 8]. Thoracoscopy in the lateral position requires a total lung block. This approach will permit a good visualization and, in the case of perioperative complications, thoracotomy will be quickly performed. Yet still the patient needs to be repositioned to the supine position for the laparoscopic phase.

The main advantage of the prone position is that it is not necessary to block the lung by double intubation. Normal intubation and a limited (7–8 mmHg) carbon dioxide (CO_2) insufflation of the right thoracic cavity is enough for an optimal visualization. Disadvantages may arise here if quick conversion is necessary, as the patient will have to be turned to the lateral position. And still a change of position from prone to supine is necessary for the laparoscopic phase. The operative techniques of thoracoscopic esophagectomy in lateral and in prone position are extensively described elsewhere [7, 8, 19]. It is essentially a three stage operation, in which a two-field lymphadenectomy is performed. It will start with the right thoracoscopy, followed by laparoscopy and the left cervical incision for the anastomosis (Figs. 9.1, 9.2, 9.3, 9.4, and 9.5). The Ivor Lewis procedure may be performed in the lateral and in the prone position, the only difference being that in the prone position the lung during the anastomosis phase will need to be blocked, due to the small thoracotomy needed for the retrieval of specimen and the introduction of circular staplers.

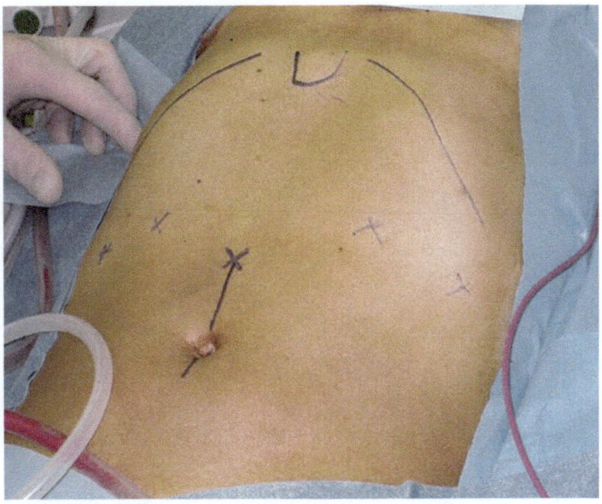

Fig. 9.6 Introduction of the trocars for laparoscopy

9.3 Thoracoscopic Esophagectomy in the Prone Position with Intrathoracic Anastomosis

In 1946, Ivor Lewis introduced a standardized approach for esophageal resection of cancer for the middle third of the esophagus [10]. This approach involves a two-stage procedure that includes a laparotomy and a right thoracotomy with thoracic anastomosis. The Ivor Lewis MIE consists of laparoscopy for gastric mobilization followed by right thoracoscopy. Thoracoscopic dissection and anastomosis can be performed in the lateral position [21] and in the prone position [22].

9.3.1 Minimally Invasive Ivor Lewis Esophagectomy in the Prone Position with Transthoracic Anastomosis

After induction of general anesthesia, the standard endotracheal intubation requires a Fogarty balloon catheter to be placed under bronchoscopy in the right bronchus (that is to be inflated only during the anastomosis phase) or else a selective double intubation follows. The patient is positioned in the supine French position.

After introduction of the trocars for laparoscopy, as depicted in Fig. 9.6 the operation starts with mobilization of the stomach and preservation

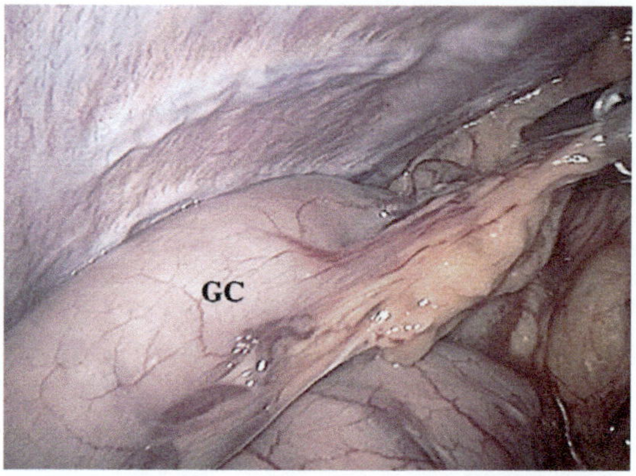

Fig. 9.7 Mobilization of the stomach and preservation of the right gastroepiploic vessels. (GC = gastric conduit)

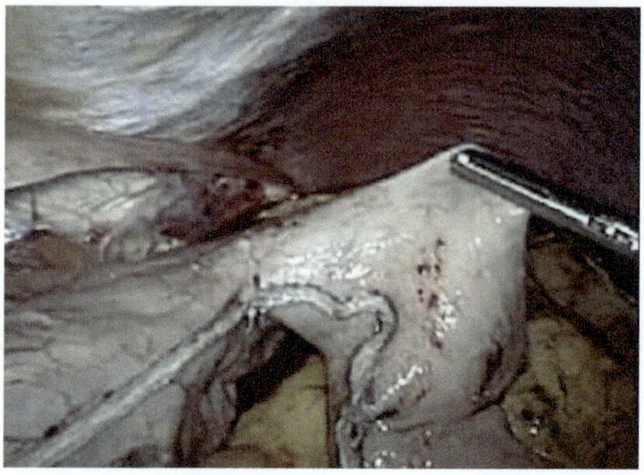

Fig. 9.9 A bridge of tissue between the gastric conduit and fundus is left for pulling the gastric conduit into the thoracic cavity

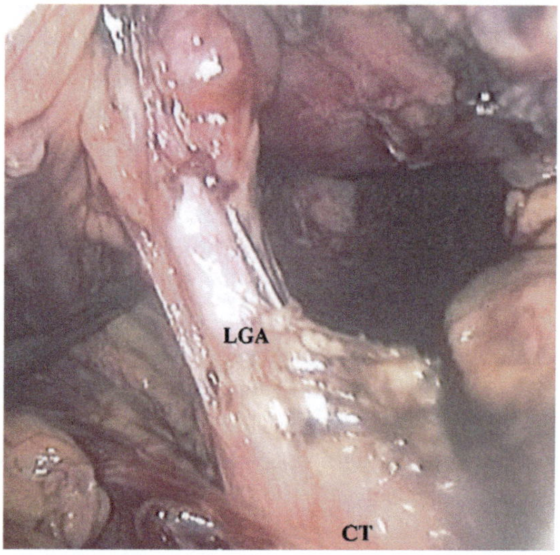

Fig. 9.8 Extensive lymphadenectomy of the celiac trunk. (LGA = left gastric artery; CT = celiac trunk)

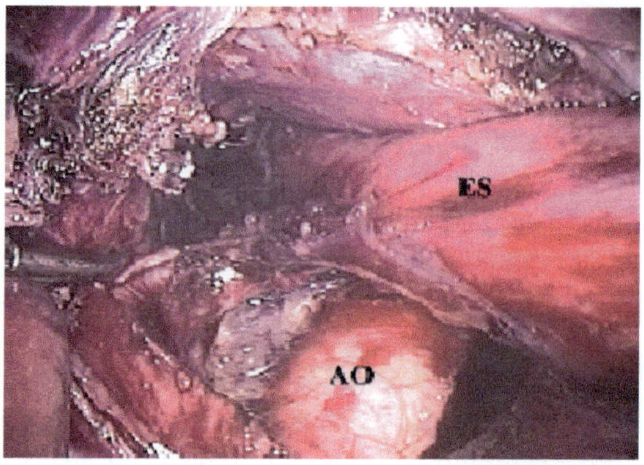

Fig. 9.10 Transhiatal dissection during Ivor Lewis, L is right lung. (AO = aorta; ES = esophagus)

of the right gastroepiploic vessels (Fig. 9.7). An extensive lymphadenectomy of the celiac trunk is performed (Fig. 9.8). A gastric conduit is created laparoscopically by means of endostaplers. A bridge of tissue between the gastric conduit and fundus is left for pulling the gastric conduit into the thoracic cavity (Fig. 9.9). Dissection of the hiatus is the last phase of the laparoscopic approach in which the hiatus is enlarged anteriorly (Fig. 9.10). A jejunostomy catheter is placed for feeding.

The patient is then positioned in the prone decubitus position (Fig. 9.1). The esophagus is dissected free with peri-esophageal tissues and lymph nodes which are removed 'en bloc' (Fig. 9.11).

The esophagus is divided at the level of the azygos arch (Fig. 9.12). The right lung is blocked with a Fogarty balloon introduced in the right bronchus. A mini-thoracotomy (5 cm) is performed at the level of the scapula tip and the ribs are spread by means of a small Finocchietto rib retractor (Fig. 9.13).

The anvil of a 25 mm circular stapler is introduced into the proximal esophagus and tightened with a purse-string suture (Fig. 9.14). The specimen is pulled into the thorax, exteriorized and resected extra-corporeally using a wound protector for the mini-thoracotomy. The stapler device is introduced into the lumen of the gastric tube and anastomosis performed in an end-to-side fashion.

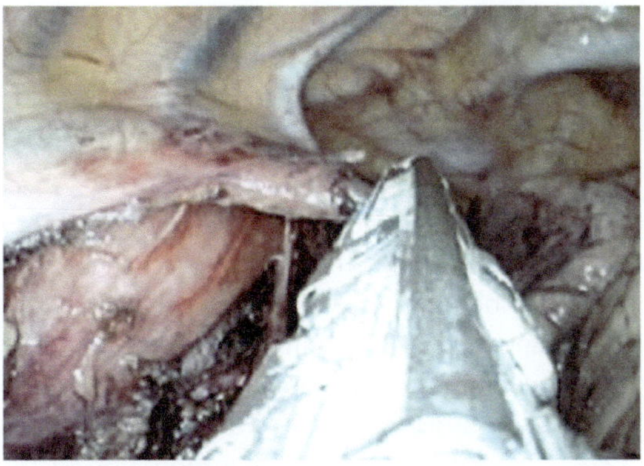

Fig. 9.11 Division of the azygos vein

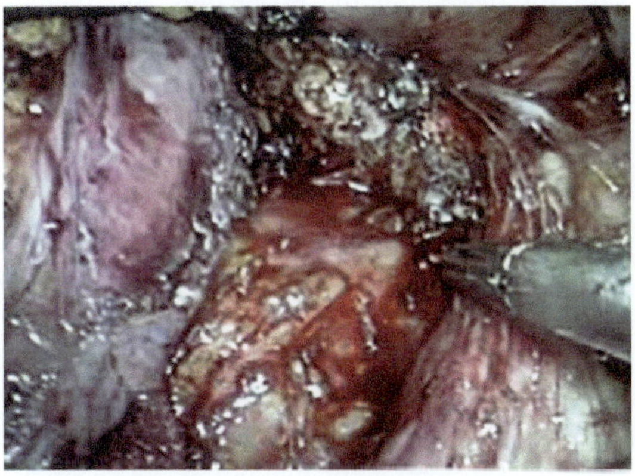

Fig. 9.12 Lymphadenectomy of the carina

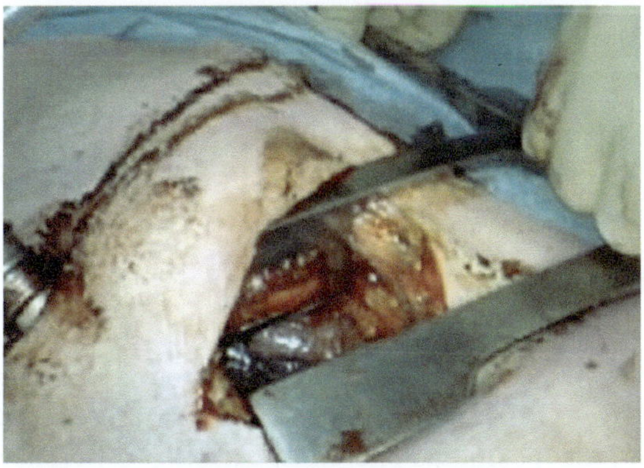

Fig. 9.13 A mini-thoracotomy (5 cm) is performed at the level of the scapula tip and the ribs are spread by means of a small Finocchietto retractor

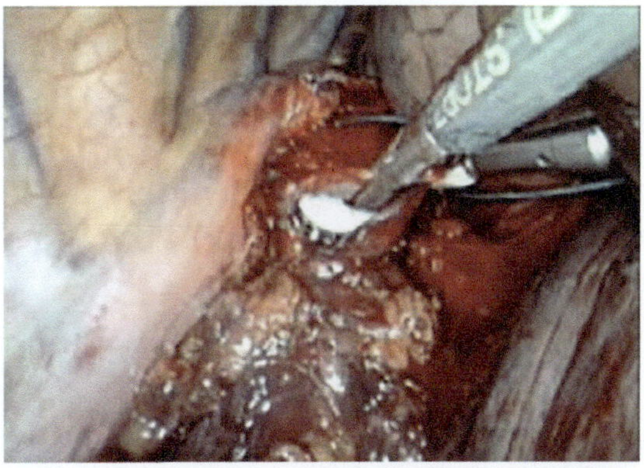

Fig. 9.14 The anvil of a 25 mm circular stapler is introduced into the proximal esophagus and tightened with a purse-string suture

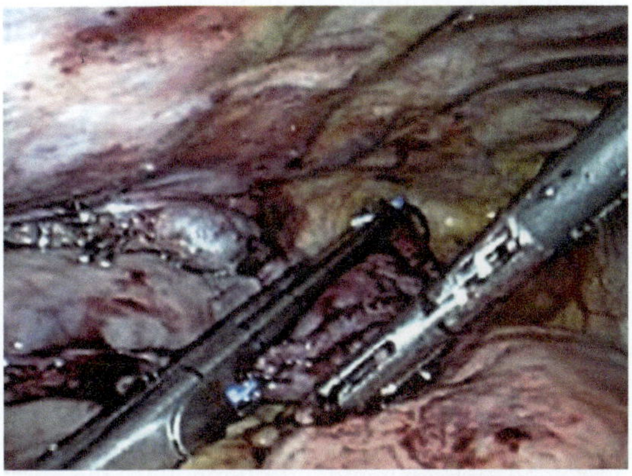

Fig. 9.15 The open part of the gastric conduit is resected by means of endostapler

The lateral loop of the gastric tube is resected by means of an endostapler (Fig. 9.15). The stapled line is reinforced with interrupted stitches (Fig. 9.16). The anastomosis is tested with methylene blue and the donuts inspected. The thoracic cavity is drained and the mini-thoracotomy closed.

9.3.2 Minimally Invasive Ivor Lewis Esophagectomy in the Prone Position with Transoral Anastomosis

An important technical development of the operation is the transoral introduction of the anvil into the proximal esophagus, as originally

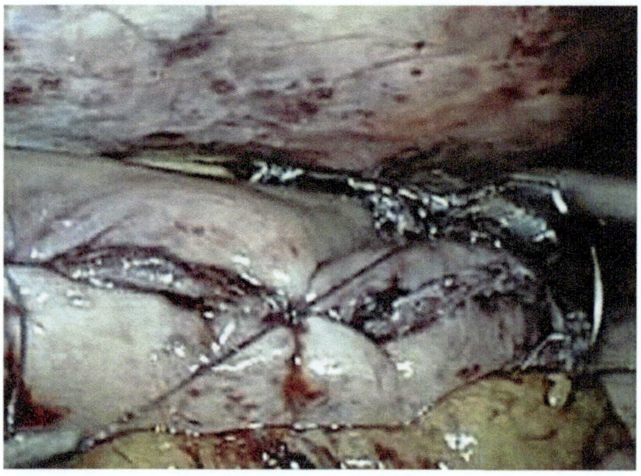

Fig. 9.16 The stapled line is reinforced with interrupted stitches

described by Wittgrove et al. in bariatric surgery [23]. Nguyen et al. described a modification of Sutton's [24] flip anvil technique in a series of ten patients [25]. A prepared pre-tilted anvil head tip attached to an oral-gastric tube is given to the anesthesiologist for oral introduction. The tilted configuration of the anvil facilitates the transoral passage. After transection of the esophagus with a linear stapler, the tube is passed transorally until it is felt within the proximal esophageal stump. A small opening at this level is made perpendicular to the staple line of the stump and the tube is advanced through it and withdrawn until the anvil is in the right position at the end of the esophageal stump. The oral-gastric tube is removed after cutting the suture attached to the anvil. The head of the anvil returns to the flat position when attached to the spike of the 25 mm circular stapler (Fig. 9.17). Campos et al. confirmed the good results using the transoral anvil technique in 37 patients with distal esophageal cancer [26]. The thoracic phase of operation was performed using a muscle-sparing mini-thoracotomy in 23 patients (62 %) and a thoracoscopic technique in 14 patients (37 %). There were no intra-operative technical failures of the anastomosis nor deaths. Five patients developed strictures (13.5 %) and all were successfully treated with endoscopic dilatations. One patient (2.7 %) had an anastomotic leak treated by re-operation and endoscopic stenting of the anastomosis.

9.4 Comparison Between Thoracoscopy in the Left Lateral Decubitus and in the Prone Position

In 1991, Dallemagne introduced the right thoracoscopic approach for esophageal cancer with total lung block, thereby mimicking the conventional approach [27]. Initial reports showed a high conversion rate to thoracotomy of 10–17 % and a respiratory morbidity ranging from 17 to 42 % [28–30]. Searching for a reduction of the conversion rate and the respiratory infection rate, Cuschieri et al. designed the thoracoscopic approach in the prone decubitus position so that total collapse of the lung was no longer necessary for dissecting the esophagus and thereby possibly reducing the rate of respiratory infections [31].

In 1949, Overholt and Woods initially described the prone decubitus position for conventional lung resection for cancer [32]. In comparison with the standard right posterolateral thoracotomy, the advantages of this approach were: (a) the attainable range of thoracic cage and diaphragmatic excursion is greater than in the side position; (b) by exposure of the posterior aspect of the hilum and esophageal area the amplitude of mediastinal swing or displacement is facilitated; (c) the weight of the lung itself allows it to fall forward; and (d) in the event of hemorrhage the blood flows away from its source, thus permitting its control with greater ease.

This approach had not been used for esophageal resection prior to the introduction of the MIE. Controversy exists as to which of the two main thoracoscopic approaches offer maximal advantages to the patient. In both approaches, a change of position from lateral or prone to supine position for the laparoscopic phase is necessary in order to finalize the procedure. Perhaps conversion to thoracotomy will be more difficult in the event of bleeding in the prone position. The most striking difference between the two approaches is the use of a complete block of the right lung by the lateral thoracoscopy (double lumen intubation) versus the limited block and normal intubation in the prone position.

Absence of one-lung ventilation may reduce arterio-venous shunt with better-preserved oxygenation [7]. In large series, MIE in the prone position seems to show a slightly better outcome regarding pulmonary infection rate compared to MIE in the lateral decubitus position (1.5 versus 7.7 %) [7, 8]. This difference may again be explained by the absence of total lung collapse in prone position [19].

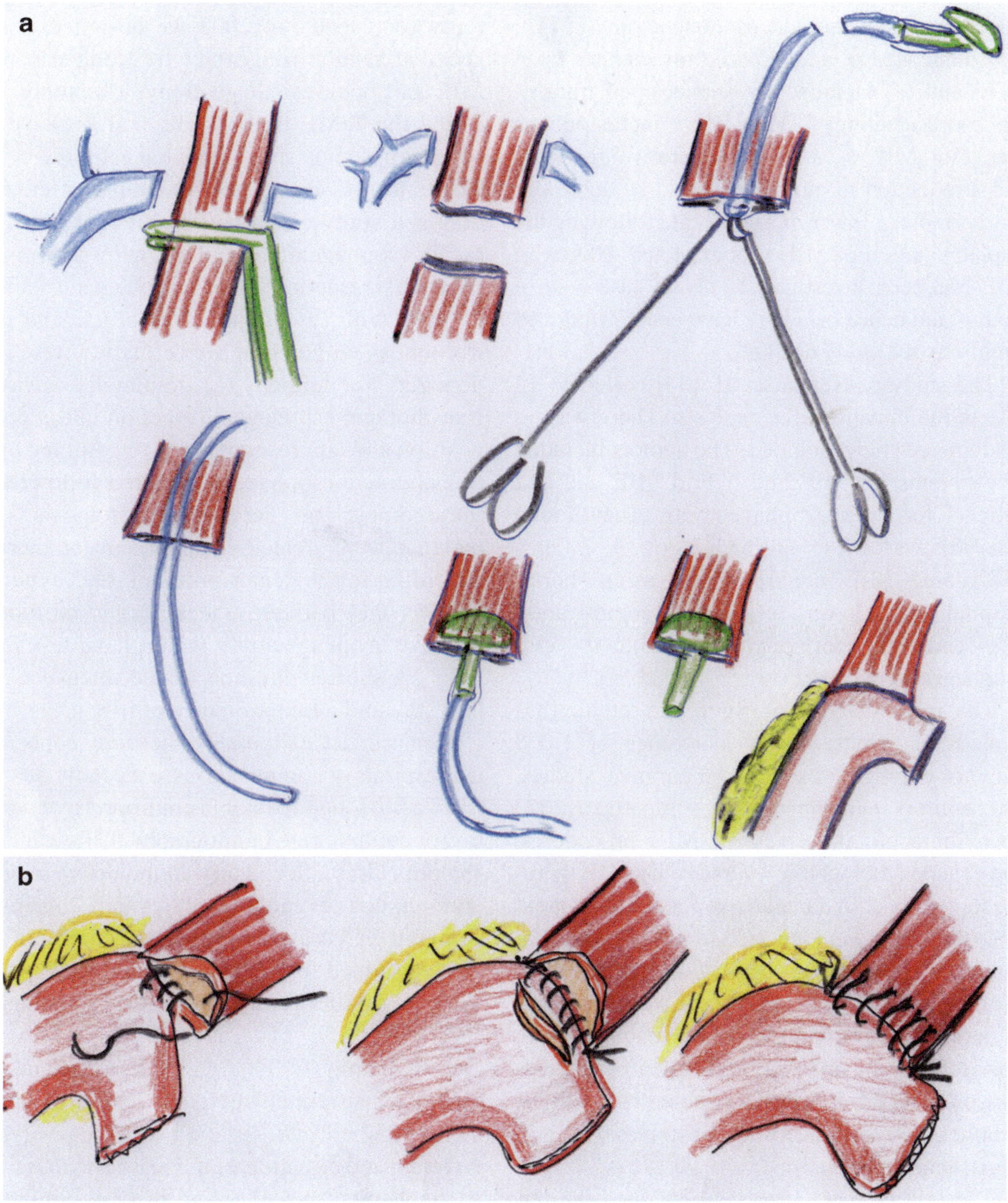

Fig. 9.17 Two possibilities of intrathoracic anastomosis, (**a**) Transoral introduction of the anvil and esophago-gastric conduit end to side anastomosis, (**b**) Manual end to side esophago-gastric conduit anastomosis

9.5 Evidence based Surgery and Outcome of the TIME trial

Three meta-analyses comparing MIE and open esophagectomy served as starting points in the quest for evidence based surgery.

Biere et al. [33] identified ten studies after a comprehensive search. Three comparative groups were created for analysis: (1) total MIE versus open transthoracic esophagectomy (TTE); (2) thoracoscopy and laparotomy versus open TTE; and (3) laparoscopy versus open transhiatal esophagectomy (THE). The conclusion was that with MIE a faster postoperative recovery and a reduction in morbidity could be achieved. Furthermore, a lower mortality rate following the implementation of MIE was expected. However, MIE had been investigated only in case control studies and hence bias may have been introduced simply by the study design.

The study of Nagpal et al. [34] collected 12 selected publications for analysis. There was no randomized study included. The authors included 672 patients for MIE and hybrid MIE and 612 patients for open esophagectomy. They found that MIE was a safe alternative option. Patients undergoing MIE could benefit from shorter hospital stay, lower respiratory complication rates and total morbidity comparable to open esophagectomy.

The meta-analysis of Sgourakis et al. [35] pooled the effects of the outcomes of 1,008 patients enrolled in eight comparative studies. The authors performed two comparisons: (1) open thoracotomy versus all MIE procedures, and (2) open thoracotomy versus only MIE thoracoscopic phase. In comparison 1, equally comparable outcomes were reported for both procedures (removed lymph nodes, 30-day mortality, 3-year survival) with the exception of the overall mortality and the anastomotic stricture that was more favourable in the open thoracotomy arm. In comparison 2, no differences were noted between the treatment arms concerning postoperative outcomes and survival.

These three meta-analyses generated the initiative for further prospective comparative or randomized-controlled trials focusing on the short term and oncological impact of MIE. Following this quest, we went on to assess the reduction of pulmonary infections and improved quality of life associated with MIE. We conducted a multicenter, randomized trial comparing open with minimally invasive esophagectomy in patients with esophageal cancer.

After a long period of practicing both the transhiatal and the thoracoscopic esophagectomy for cancer, in 2008 we designed a prospective randomized study for comparison of MIE and open esophagectomy. The study was called the TIME trial (Traditional Invasive vs. Minimally invasive Esophagectomy). The TIME trial is a prospective, multicenter, randomized study comparing traditional transthoracic esophageal resection with minimally invasive resection for esophageal cancer. Patients with resectable intrathoracic and gastroesophageal junction Siewert type I were randomized for either: (a) minimally invasive transthoracic esophageal resection in the prone position and laparoscopy, or (b) traditional open transthoracic esophageal resection followed by intrathoracic or cervical anastomosis. All patients were treated by neoadjuvant therapy according to the center protocol. Our hypothesis was that patients undergoing a minimally invasive esophagectomy would have less morbidity, a shorter duration of the intensive care unit stay and a better quality of life.

The primary endpoint of the study concerned the respiratory complications, especially postoperative bronchopneumonia confirmed by chest X ray, or computarized tomography (CT) scan, and sputum culture. Secondary endpoints were operation-related events, complications, intensive care unit (ICU) and hospital stay, quality of life as determined by questionnaires Short Form (SF)-36 and European Organization for Research and Treatment of Cancer Quality of life Questionnaire (EORTC C30-OES18), and the quality of specimen resected (length of specimen, number and location of lymph nodes resected, and circumferential resection margins). Also, hospital mortality and readmissions were recorded. Furthermore, survival analysis will be performed.

The power of the study was calculated according to the published literature and our experience at the VU University Medical Center, Amsterdam, Netherlands.

We took into consideration that a difference in respiratory infections of 28 % can be found between the traditional open procedure (57 %) and the MIE procedure (29 %) [6–8]. To demonstrate this difference of 28 %, using an alpha=0.5 and beta=0.80, two groups of 48 patients were required. Estimating that approximately 20 % of the eligible patients would not undergo the allocated intervention (e.g. metastases during neoadjuvant therapy, irresectable tumors), approximately 60 patients per group were asked to participate.

We then hypothesized that the lower incidence of pulmonary infections found in the MIE group could be explained by several factors, which taken all together might reduce the development of atelectasis. We held the following suppositions. Use of the prone position in comparison with the open thoracotomy in lateral position could be one of the underlying factors for prevention of atelectasis. In contrast with the lateral decubitus position, in prone position the mediastinum hangs in its usual midposition and the chest and abdomen are free of compression [32]. A second advantage may be the avoidance of a total collapse of the lung during MIE in prone position. The right lung is partially collapsed by gravity and by CO_2 insufflation to a maximum pressure of 8 mmHg. This permits an optimal visualization of the mediastinum with preserved ventilation and oxygenation in contrast to the required one-lung ventilation for open esophagectomy [36, 37]. Absence of one-lung ventilation reduces arterio-venous shunt with better preserved oxygenation [7]. Another possible underlying factor for the higher rate of pulmonary infection in open eophagectomy may be the thoracotomy wound itself. Not only does the development of atelectasis as result of the totally collapsed lung play a role, but also the postoperative discomfort from the thoracotomy wound causes an increased rate of pulmonary infections [38]. All these factors could explain the important advantages of thoracoscopy in prone position in comparison with the standard posterolateral right thoracotomy. The rate of pulmonary infection in the open esophagectomy is clearly lower than the rate used for the sample size calculation. Current preoperative programs – including physiotherapy, psychological assistance and adequate nutritional support – may explain this substantial decrease [39].

Between June 2009 and March 2011, 144 patients became eligible for randomization. Of these, 29 were excluded for various reasons. A total of 115 patients underwent randomization in five centers (VU University Medical Center and the Academic Medical Center both in Amsterdam, Netherlands; the Canisius Wilhelmina Ziekenhuis in Nijmegen, Netherlands; Hospital Universitario dr. Josep Trueta in Girona, Spain; and IRCCS Policlinico San Donato at the University of Milano, in Milan, Italy). Finally 56 patients were analyzed in the open group and 59 in the MIE group [40].

The pulmonary infection rate within the first 2 weeks was 29 % (16 patients) in the open group and 9 % (5 patients) in the MIE group, $p=0.005$. The overall hospital incidence of pulmonary infections was 34 % (19 patients) in the open group and 12 % (7 patients) in the MIE group, $p=0.005$. A likely explanation for the lower incidence of pulmonary infections in the MIE group is that in the prone decubitus the mediastinum is not displaced; a second advantage is the partial collapse of the lung during the MIE (double lung ventilation) that permits optimal visualization of mediastinum with preserved ventilation and oxygenation; a third factor may be the absence of the thoracotomy wound itself. All factors together could explain the better outcome with MIE.

In addition, MIE preserved the quality of life better than the open approach. After 6 weeks all the questionnaires (SF 36, EORTC C30 and the specific OES 18 questionnaire) showed better results in the MIE group than in the open group.

Hospital stay was significantly shorter in the MIE group (14 versus 11 days, $p=0.044$), reflecting a faster postoperative recovery. Other postoperative data including pathology parameters, major postoperative complications (anastomotic leakage, 7 % in the open and 12 % in the

MIE group, p=0.390) and mortality (1.8 versus 3.4 %) were not significantly different. Interestingly, the vocal cord paralysis rate was 14 % in the open group and only 2 % in the MIE group, p=0.012. Pneumatic dissection by CO_2 from the thoracic cavity into the neck can simplify the dissection in the neck and reduce the risk of recurrent nerve lesions.

In conclusion, the randomized TIME trial comparing open esophagectomy for cancer with minimally invasive esophagectomy on the short term shows that MIE results in a lower incidence of pulmonary infections, a shorter hospital stay, and a better short-term quality of life without compromise of the quality of the resected specimen.

Key Points

- Pulmonary complications are common after esophagectomy
- Minimally invasive esophagectomy has the potential to reduce morbidity and improve quality of life
- The thoracoscopic approach in the prone position with two-lung ventilation has resulted in a significant reduction of pulmonary complications and an improved short-term quality of life

References

1. Jemal A, Bray F, Center MM, Ferlay J, Ward E, Forman D (2011) Global cancer statistics. CA Cancer J Clin 61:69–90
2. Parkin DM, Pisani P, Ferlay J (1999) Global cancer statistics. CA Cancer J Clin 49:33–64
3. Enzinger PC, Mayer RJ (2003) Esophageal cancer. N Engl J Med 349:2241–2252
4. Sjoquist KM, Burmeister BH, Smithers BM, Zalcberg JR, Simes RJ, Barbour A, Gebski V (2011) Survival after neoadjuvant chemotherapy or chemoradiotherapy for resectable oesophageal carcinoma: an updated meta-analysis. Lancet Oncol 12:681–692
5. Scheepers JJ, Mulder CJ, van der Peet DL, Meijer S, Cuesta MA (2006) Minimally invasive oesophageal resection for distal oesophageal cancer; a review of literature. Scand J Gastroenterol (41 suppl): 123–134
6. Hulscher JBF, van Sandwick JW, de Boer AG et al (2002) Extended transthoracic resection compared with limited transhiatal resection for adenocarcinoma of the esophagus. N Engl J Med 347:1662–1669
7. Palanivelu C, Prakash A, Senthilkumar R, Senthilnathan P, Parthasarthi R, Rajan S, Venkatachlam S (2006) Minimally invasive esophagectomy: thoracoscopic mobilization of the esophagus and mediastinal lymphadenectomy in prone position – experience of 130 patients. J Am Coll Surg 203:7–16
8. Luketich JD, Alvelo-Rivera M, Bunaventura PO et al (2003) Minimally invasive esophagectomy: outcomes in 222 patients. Ann Surg 238:486–494
9. MacKeown McKeown KC (1976) Total three-stage oesophagectomy for cancer of the oesophagus. Br J Surg 63:259–262
10. Lewis I (1946) The surgical treatment of carcinoma of the oesophagus: with special reference to a new operation for growths of the middle third. Br J Surg 34:18–31
11. Djary T, Metcalfe C, Avery KN, Lagergren P, Blazeby JM (2010) Prognostic value of changes in health-related quality of life scores during curative treatment for esophagogastric cancer. J Clin Oncol 1(28):1666–1670
12. Orringer MB, Sloan H (1978) Esophagectomy without thoracotomy. J Thorac Cardiovasc Surg 76:643–654
13. Scheepers JJ, Veenhof AA, van der Peet DL, van Groeningen C, Mulder C, Meijer S, Cuesta MA (2008) Laparoscopic transhiatal resection for malignancies of the distal esophagus: outcome of the first 50 resected patients. Surgery 143:278–285
14. Akiyama H (1988) Cardinals in the regional lymph node dissection in surgery of thoracic esophageal cancer. In: Siewert JR, Holscher AH (eds) Diseases of the esophagus. Springer, Berlin, p 416
15. Siewert JR, Stein HJ, Feith M (2006) Adenocarcinoma of the esophago-gastric junction. Scand J Surg 95: 260–269
16. Gebski V, Burmeister B, Smithers BM et al (2007) Survival benefits from neoadjuvant chemoradiotherapy or chemotherapy in oesophageal carcinoma: a meta-analysis. Lancet Oncol 8:226–234
17. Cunningham D, Allum WH, Stenning SP et al (2006) Peroperative chemotherapy versus surgery alone for resectable gastroesophageal cancer. N Engl J Med 355:11–20
18. van Hagen P, Hulshof MC, van Lanschot JJ et al. Preoperative chemoradiotherapy for esophageal or junctional cancer. N Eng J Med 2012;366:2074–84
19. Cuesta MA, Scheepers JJG, Oosterhuis W et al (2010) Thoracoscopic esophageal resection for cancer in prone decubitus position: operative technique. In: Puntambekar S, Cuesta MA (eds) Atlas of minimally invasive surgery in esophageal carcinoma. Springer, Dordrecht/New York, pp 149–169
20. Biere SSAY, Maas KW, Cuesta MA, van der Peet DL (2011) Cervical or thoracic anastomosis after esophagectomy for cancer: a systematic review and meta-analysis. Dig Surg 28:29–35

21. Bizekis C, Kent MS, Luketich JD et al (2006) Initial experience with minimally invasive Ivor Lewis esophagectomy. Ann Thorac Surg 82:402–406
22. Cadiere GB, Dapri G, Himpens J, Fodderie L, Rajan A (2010) Ivor Lewis esophagectomy with manual esogastric anastomosis by thoracoscopy in prone position and laparoscopy. Surg Endosc 24:1482–1485
23. Wittgrove AC, Clark WG, Tremblay LJ (2004) Laparoscopic gastric bypass, Roux-en-Y: preliminary report of five cases. Obes Surg 4:353–357
24. Sutton CD, White SA, Marshall LJ, Berry DP, Veith PS (2002) Endoscopic-assisted intrathoracic oesophagectomy without thoracotomy for tumours of the lower oesophagus and cardia. Eur J Surg Oncol 28:46–48
25. Nguyen NT, Hinojosa MW, Smith BR, Gray J, Reavis KM (2008) Thoracoscopic construction of an intrathoracic esophagogastric anastomosis using a circular stapler: transoral placement of the anvil. Ann Thorac Surg 86:989–993
26. Campos MC, Jablons D, Brown LM, Ramirez RM, Rabl C, Theodore P (2010) A safe reproducible anastomotic technique for minimally invasive Ivor Lewis esophagectomy: the circular-stapled anastomosis with the trans-oral anvil. Eur J Cardiothorac Surg 37:1421–1426
27. Dallemagne B, Weerts JM, Jehaes C (1993) Thoracoscopic oesophageal resection. In: Cuesta MA, Nagy AG (eds) Minimally invasive surgery in gastrointestinal cancer. Churchill Livingstone, Edinburgh/New York, pp 59–68
28. Azagra JS, Ceuterick M, Goergen M et al (1993) Thoracoscopy in oesophagectomy for oesophageal cancer. Br J Surg 80:320–321
29. Gossot D, Fourquier P, Celerier M (1993) Thoracoscopic oesophagectomy: technique and initial results. Ann Thorac Surg 56:667–670
30. McAnena OJ, Rogers J, Williams NS (1994) Right thoracoscopically assisted oesophagectomy for cancer. Br J Surg 81:236–238
31. Cuschieri A (1994) Thoracoscopic subtotal oesophagectomy. Endosc Surg Allied Technol 2:21–25
32. Overholt RH, Woods FM (1947) The prone position in thoracic surgery. J Int Coll Surg 10:216
33. Biere SSAY, Cuesta MA, van der Peet DL (2009) Minimally invasive versus open esophagectomy for cancer: a systematic review and meta-analysis. Minerva Chir 64:121–133
34. Nagpal K, Ahmed K, Vats A et al (2010) Is minimally invasive surgery beneficial in the management of esophageal cancer? A meta-analysis. Surg Endosc 24:1621–1629
35. Sgourakis G, Gockel I, Radtke A et al (2010) Minimally invasive versus open esophagectomy: meta-analysis of outcomes. Dig Dis Sci 55:3031–3040
36. Yatabe T, Kitagawa H, Yamashita K, Akimori T, Hanazaki K, Yokoyama M (2010) Better postoperative oxygenation in thoracoscopic esophagectomy in prone positioning. J Anesth 24:803–806
37. Fabian T, Martin J, Katigbak M, McKelvey AA, Federico JA (2008) Thoracoscopic esophageal mobilization during minimally invasive esophagectomy: a head-to-head comparison of prone versus lateral decubitus positions. Surg Endosc 22:2485–2491
38. Grogan EL, Jones DR (2008) VATS lobectomy is better than open thoracotomy: what is the evidence for short-term outcomes? Thorac Surg Clin 18:249–258
39. Biere SSAY, Maas KW, Bonavina L et al (2011) Traditional invasive vs. minimally invasive esophagectomy: a multi-center, randomized trial. BMC Surg 11:2
40. Biere SSAY, van Berge Henegouwen M, Maas KW, Bonavina L, Rosman C, Roig Garcia J, Gisbertz SS, Klinkenbijl JHG, Hollmann MW, de Lange ESM, Bonjer HJ, van der Peet DL, Cuesta MA. Minimally invasive versus open oesophagectomy for cancer: a multicentre, open label, randomised controlled trial, Lancet 2012;379:1887–92

10 Limited Versus Extended Lymphadenectomy

S. Michael Griffin and Shajahan Wahed

The main aims of surgery for esophageal cancer resection are to prolong survival, achieve long-term cure and minimize the chances of locoregional disease recurrence. The primary tumor and surrounding tissues including the relevant lymphatic drainage fields are therefore removed during esophagectomy with extended lymphadenectomy. The resected specimen provides the most accurate staging for depth, extent and invasion of the primary tumor as well as information about any lymph node involvement for prognostic purposes. The surgical approach used must achieve these goals whilst ensuring low morbidity, low mortality and maintaining an optimal quality of life. The extent of the lymphadenectomy at the time of esophagectomy potentially impacts on all these aspects.

Proponents of limited lymphadenectomy hold the view that lymph nodes positive for metastases merely reflect the presence of systemic disease, and so removing more lymph nodes will not affect survival. The converse opinion is that the presence of lymph node metastases does not imply the presence of widespread systemic disease, particularly in patients with a limited positive burden, and so formal removal of the lymph nodes is necessary for a curative procedure. The controversy regarding the value of an extended lymphadenectomy persists due to the heterogeneous nature of the published literature. Much of the evidence has to be extrapolated from studies comparing transhiatal and transthoracic approaches. Although these are two distinct surgical procedures, the predominant difference is the extent of the lymphadenectomy. Studies have combined adenocarcinoma and squamous cell cancers in analyses, despite growing evidence that the behaviour of these two histological entities is different. Such studies have also compared two-field with three-field lymphadenectomy, both of which can be considered as extended procedures. Further questions arise when one considers whether the same lymphadenectomy should be applied to all patients undergoing esophagectomy irrespective of the stage of disease.

10.1 Definitions of the Extent of Lymphadenectomy

It is crucial to have an understanding of the correct definitions relating to the operative procedure and lymphadenectomy [1]. The literature contains

S.M. Griffin (✉) • S. Wahed
Northern Oesophago-Gastric Cancer Unit,
Royal Victoria Infirmary, Queen Victoria Road,
Newcastle upon Tyne, NE1 4LP, UK
e-mail: michael.griffin@nuth.nhs.uk

L. Bonavina (ed.), *Innovation in Esophageal Surgery*,
DOI 10.1007/978-88-470-2469-4_10, © Springer-Verlag Italia 2012

too many publications that fail clearly to specify the extent of the lymphadenectomy. A limited lymphadenectomy is defined as the removal of the peritumoral lymph nodes and lymph nodes immediately adjacent to the resected part of the esophagus or stomach. An extended or radical lymphadenectomy in the context of an esophageal resection refers to the systematic removal of all lymph nodes within at least the upper abdominal and mediastinal fields (Fig. 10.1). Extended lymphadenectomy can be subdivided into two-field or three-field depending on whether lymph nodes in the cervical region are systematically removed. A true extended two-field lymphadenectomy should include resection of all the nodal stations in the mediastinum. In practice however there is a significant risk of recurrent laryngeal nerve damage with formal dissection of the left recurrent laryngeal nodal chain, so these nodes are often not resected in lower-third adenocarcinomas.

The term 'en bloc' is frequently used in the literature. The correct use of this term simply refers to the removal of the primary cancer and adjacent nodal tissue as one specimen. In practice, en bloc resection is an extended lymphadenectomy, whether this is two-field or three-field.

The different surgical approaches to an esophagectomy, whether open or minimally invasive, can be used to obtain a limited or an exteneded lymphadenectomy, as wished. For instance transhiatal esophagectomy in the majority of cases involves a limited lymphadenectomy, as the complete field of mediastinal lymph nodes is not resected and often only a very limited abdominal nodal dissection is performed [2]. Nevertheless radical transhiatal resections are possible for lower third esophageal cancers [3]. The single incision left thoraco-abdominal approach allows access to the more of mediastinal lymph nodes but an extended two-field lymphadenectomy can only be achieved using both a laparotomy and right thoracotomy.

A 2-stage esophagectomy with extended two-field lymphadenectomy involves mobilization of the stomach via an upper midline incision with dissection of all the upper abdominal lymph nodes highlighted in Fig. 10.1 and division of the left gastric vein and artery at origin, with preservation of the right gastric and right gastro-epiploic arteries. The right posterolateral thoracotomy permits division of the azygos vein, en bloc dissection of the thoracic duct and mediastinal lymph node fields and the esophagus. The stomach is brought up into the chest before removal of

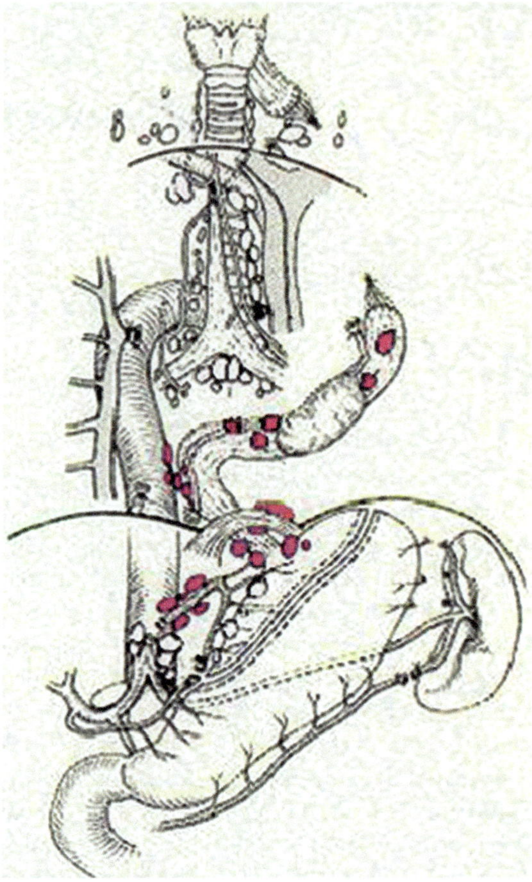

Fig. 10.1 Lymph nodes removed in an extended two-field lymphadenectomy

Abdominal	Mediastinal
Celiac	Paratracheal
Common hepatic	Carinal
Left gastric	Right bronchial
Splenic	Left bronchial
Lesser curve	Middle paraesophageal
Right paracardial	Lower paraesophageal
Left paracardial	Para-aortic
	Thoracic duct

the esophagus with the lymph node fields and creation of the esophago-gastric anastomosis [1].

Complete removal of all mediastinal nodes or an extended three-field lymphadenectomy involves removal of the cervical lymph nodes as part of a 3-stage procedure.

10.2 Optimal Staging

The importance of numbers with respect to nodes is reflected in the *TNM Classification of Malignant Tumors*, 7th edition. Nodal stage is subdivided according to whether 0, 1–2, 3–6 or more than 6 lymph nodes are positive. This influences the overall stage grouping for an individual, which in turn informs prognosis [4, 5]. It is therefore logical to appreciate that by removing more lymph nodes with an extended lymphadenectomy, a more accurate lymph node status will be obtained. Considerable advances have been made with preoperative imaging including thoracic and abdominal computed tomography, endoscopic and neck ultrasound, and positron emission tomography but as yet even combinations of these modalities are not accurate enough to predict the nodal status for all cases.

A prospective study evaluating transthoracic esophagectomy for adenocarcinoma found that the extended lymphadenectomy upstaged the disease in 17 out of 74 (23 %) cases [6]. The same group demonstrated a 22 % mediastinal lymph node metastasis rate in patients with type II esophago-gastric junction adenocarcinoma undergoing extended transthoracic esophagectomy [7]. These are nodes that would not normally be removed by techniques incorporating limited lymphadenectomy. One retrospective study of 336 patients, with adenocarcinoma as the predominant histological subtype, has suggested that the minimum number of lymph nodes required for accurate staging in esophageal cancer is 18 [8]. Akiyama et al. have previously shown that for squamous cell carcinoma, extended three-field lymphadenectomy upstaged patients compared to those having a thoraco-abdominal procedure with two-field lymphadenectomy [9]. Another prospective observational study examining both adenocarcinoma and squamous cell cancer found that 30 % of patients were upstaged when a three-field node dissection was performed [10].

Accurate nodal staging is important as the extent of nodal involvement is of prognostic significance in esophageal adenocarcinoma and squamous cell carcinoma including in those patients who have received neoadjuvant therapy. Not only does the absolute number of positive lymph nodes affect prognosis, but the ratio of positive lymph nodes to removed lymph nodes has also been shown to influence survival [11, 12]. Siewert et al. showed in their study of 186 patients with squamous cell cancer undergoing en bloc esophagectomy that the ratio of positive lymph nodes was second only to achieving a complete (R0) resection as the most important factor in prognosis [11]. The true node ratio can only be calculated if an extended lymphadenectomy is performed.

It is vital to appreciate the widespread variation in the handling of resected specimens between centers. Lymph node yields will inevitably differ between patients but how the specimen is dissected will impact on the ability of pathologist to identify and examine lymph nodes. The optimal method is for the operating surgeon to dissect out individual nodal groups and provide these as separate specimens for the pathologist to examine. Additional consideration needs to be given to lymph node negative patients. Sampling errors when nodes are processed can never be completely removed and will depend on the number of sections processed for each node. There is no current standardization of histopathology processing. Further uncertainty continues to exist concerning the long-term significance of micrometastases and isolated tumor cells within lymph nodes.

10.3 Enhanced Locoregional Control

Evidence has existed for many years now that in the absence of any formal lymphadenectomy, locoregional recurrence rates after esophagectomy are high [13]. A randomized controlled study for adenocarcinoma showed that nodal harvest from a transthoracic approach to esophagectomy was almost double that from a transhiatal approach (means 31±14 versus 16±9) [14]. This Dutch study demonstrated that in patients with a limited number of positive lymph nodes (1–8) there was a 17 % lower locoregional recurrence rate in patients operated on via the transthoracic approach. This translated into a staggering 41 % locoregional disease-free survival advantage at 5 years in these patients with a limited nodal burden [15].

Locoregional recurrence rates in non-randomized studies for adenocarcinoma and squamous cell carcinoma approaching 40 % following transhiatal resection have been reported [13]. This compares to lower rates of 27 % following radical two-field lymphadenectomy in a separate study; for adenocarcinoma the rate was even lower at 19 % [16]. An impressive locoregional recurrence of just 10 % (local recurrence was just 1 %) following radical en bloc dissection for adenocarcinoma has been reported from Hagen et al. in the US [17]. Very few of the locoregional recurrences in these studies were cervical, suggesting that there is minimal potential gain from a three-field lymphadenectomy over two-field in all cases [16, 17].

10.4 Long-Term Survival

There is clear evidence that achieving a R0 resection is associated with better long-term outcomes. To date there are few randomized trials comparing limited and extended lymphadenectomy, and all those existing are underpowered [18–20]. The Dutch study compared extended transthoracic resection with limited transhiatal resection for esophageal and esophago-gastric junction adenocarcinoma [14, 15]. The results suggest an improved survival from transthoracic resection at 5 years and beyond. The 5-year data demonstrated a 14 % improved survival for patients with type 1 esophageal adenocarcinoma treated with transthoracic resection [15].

A further striking observation from this study was that for patients with a limited nodal burden of between 1 and 8 positive lymph nodes there was a 20 % 5-year survival advantage following transthoracic resection. The logical explanation for these observations would be that removing more nodes in the context of definite node-negative disease would not affect survival. Similarly, the presence of extensive lymph node metastases might simply reflect the more advanced nature of the disease possibly with occult systemic metastases, in which scenario an extended lymphadenectomy would not affect long-term survival. One large study has shown that the incidence of systemic disease within 5 years is 93 % in patients who have eight or more positive lymph nodes [21]. It must be remembered that determining whether a patient is indeed node-negative can only be achieved if sufficient nodes are removed and examined.

Short-term outcomes also need to be considered when comparing the extent of lymphadenectomy. The risks of pulmonary complications and of chyle leaks following extended lymphadenectomy were higher in the Dutch randomized study [14]. One would expect these observations given the thoracotomy and increased radicality of the surgery but it is important to note that there was no difference in the in-hospital mortality.

Several recent large series provide additional evidence in support of radical lymphadenectomy. These highlight the number of lymph nodes removed as being an independent predictor of survival: there is a minimum number of lymph nodes that should be removed and the more nodes that are removed the better the overall survival. In a 9-center prospective international study involving 2,303 patients, none of whom received neoadjuvant or adjuvant treatment, survival according to numbers of lymph nodes removed in groups of ten nodes was analysed [22]. With increasing numbers of nodes resected a significant increase in survival at 5 years was evident. A resected number of 23 lymph nodes appeared to be the threshold above which a survival advantage was evident. This was true across all stages of disease. The survival advantage was independent of the actual number of lymph node metastases. The number of nodes removed was therefore the third most important prognostic factor after the number of nodes involved and the tumor depth.

This study illustrated that achieving resection of this threshold of 23 lymph nodes in most patients was attainable only with esophagectomy with extended lymphadenectomy. Furthermore, resections with extended lymphadenectomy achieved a 14 % 5-year survival advantage even when the apparent threshold harvest of 23 nodes was attained.

The Worldwide Esophageal Cancer Collaboration characterized the relationship between survival and extent of lymphadenectomy, and from this defined the optimal lymphadenectomy [23]. A total of 4,627 patients who had esophagectomy alone for adenocarcinoma or squamous cell cancer were identified. The results showed that greater extent of lymphadenectomy was associated with increased survival. This included cases that were negative for lymph node metastases but were moderately or poorly-differentiated cancers. The groups where survival was not influenced by the extent of lymphadenectomy were the extremes of carcinoma *in situ*, well-differentiated cancers in node-negative patients and patients who had more than seven positive lymph nodes. This study also identified that the optimum lymphadenectomy increased as the histopathological depth of the primary tumor (T stage) increased. If T stage and grade cannot be accurately determined pre-operatively the recommendations, based on this study, were to resect 30 or more nodes to optimize 5-year survival. This can only be achieved via extended lymphadenectomy. As with other multicenter studies there was no standardized protocol for the surgery, lymphadenectomy or pathological processing but the number of cases included was impressive and so the results cannot be dismissed.

A large study from the US population-based Surveillance Epidemiology and End Results (SEER) cancer registry, that is designed to capture a representative sample of the US population, analysed survival according to stratification of numbers of lymph nodes examined [24]. Patients who had 30 or more lymph nodes examined had significantly better long-term survival.

One recent retrospective single center study of 264 patients noted that survival following esophagectomy improved as the number of resected nodes increased. This was particularly true for patients who had lymph node metastases [25]. The majority of other studies and anecdotal evidence support extended lymphadenectomy [16, 26, 27]. There are a few studies that have failed to demonstrate a survival improvement [28, 29].

In stage 3 disease there have been reports of improved survival following 3-stage procedures with cervical lymphadenectomy when compared to 2-stage esophagectomy [30, 31]. Nevertheless the value of 3-stage procedures for lower-third esophageal cancers, particularly adenocarcinoma, remains unproven. Without pre-operative evidence of neck node involvement a routine three-field lymphadenectomy in patients is not recommended in the Western world. Indeed the presence of potential neck nodes in adenocarcinoma might signal the presence of systemic disease.

10.5 Lymphadenectomy in Early Disease

Recent evidence has been published showing that the risk of lymph node metastasis in mucosal cancers is minimal [32, 33]. These patients with mucosal disease might not gain additional benefit from the extended lymphadenectomy so may be suitable for limited resection with limited lymphadenectomy or even endoscopic mucosal resection [34]. However results with radical surgery in specialist centers in these patients are so good that any less radical techniques must be cautiously introduced and the outcomes widely reported to ensure comparable results. Submucosal disease should still be treated with surgery and an extended lymphadenectomy, as the lymph node metastasis rate is appreciable for all levels of submucosal involvement and current staging investigations are not sensitive or specific enough to accurately identify nodal disease in these patients [32].

Endoscopic mucosal resection as a staging/diagnostic procedure could potentially identify patients with unifocal, intramucosal disease in whom surgery can be avoided. Research into sentinel lymph node localization for esophageal cancer has shown this to be feasible and accurate

[35]. Further research into this exciting field and the development of other imaging modalities might prove beneficial in accurately identifying patients suitable for limited lymphadenectomy.

Conclusion

There needs to be worldwide agreement on the definitions used to describe esophageal resections and specifically the extent of lymphadenectomy. Extended two-field lymphadenectomy performed by experienced operators currently offers patients a long-term survival advantage. Three-field lymphadenectomy should be reserved for upper third tumors. Extended lymphadenectomy should remain the gold standard until newer staging investigations can accurately predict lymph node status and identify patients potentially suitable for more limited resections.

Key Points

- Standardized definitions of lymphadenectomy need to be clearly reported in publications
- Extended lymphadenectomy improves the accuracy of disease staging, reduces locoregional recurrence and increases chances of cure
- The advantages of extended lymphadenectomy are greatest in patients with a limited positive nodal burden
- Variability and uncertainty exists in the histopathological processing of lymph nodes
- Justification for a limited lymphadenectomy can only emerge following the development of more accurate staging

References

1. Griffin SM, Raimes SA (2009) Oesophagogastric surgery, 4th edn. Saunders/Elsevier, Edinburgh, pp 91–115
2. Orringer MB, Marshall B, Chang AC, Lee J, Pickens A, Lau CL (2007) Two thousand transhiatal esophagectomies: changing trends, lessons learned. Ann Surg 246:363–372
3. Alderson D, Courtney SP, Kennedy RH (1994) Radical transhiatal oesophagectomy under direct vision. Br J Surg 81:404–407
4. Edge SB, Byrd DR, Compton CC, Fritz AG, Greene FL, Trotti A (2009) AJCC cancer staging manual, 7th edn. Springer, New York, pp 103–115
5. Rice TW, Blackstone EH, Rusch VW (2010) 7th edition of the AJCC cancer staging manual: esophagus and esophagogastric junction. Ann Surg Oncol 17: 1721–1724
6. Hulscher JB, Van Sandick JW, Offerhaus GJ, Tilanus HW, Obertop H, Van Lanschot JJ (2001) Prospective analysis of the diagnostic yield of extended en bloc resection for adenocarcinoma of the oesophagus or gastric cardia. Br J Surg 88:715–719
7. Lagarde SM, Cense HA, Hulscher JB, Tilanus HW, Ten Kate FJ, Obertop H et al (2005) Prospective analysis of patients with adenocarcinoma of the gastric cardia and lymph node metastasis in the proximal field of the chest. Br J Surg 92:1404–1408
8. Rizk N, Venkatraman E, Park B, Flores R, Bains MS, Rusch V (2006) The prognostic importance of the number of involved lymph nodes in esophageal cancer: implications for revisions of the American Joint Committee on Cancer staging system. J Thorac Cardiovasc Surg 132:1374–1381
9. Akiyama H, Tsurumaru M, Udagawa H, Kajiyama Y (1994) Radical lymph node dissection for cancer of the thoracic esophagus. Ann Surg 220:364–372
10. Altorki N, Kent M, Ferrara C, Port J (2002) Three-field lymph node dissection for squamous cell and adenocarcinoma of the esophagus. Ann Surg 236: 177–183
11. Siewert JR, Fink U, Beckurts KT, Roder JD (1994) Surgery of squamous cell carcinoma of the esophagus. Ann Oncol 5(Suppl 3):1–7
12. Mariette C, Piessen G, Briez N, Triboulet JP (2008) The number of metastatic lymph nodes and the ratio between metastatic and examined lymph nodes are independent prognostic factors in esophageal cancer regardless of neoadjuvant chemoradiation or lymphadenectomy extent. Ann Surg 247:365–371
13. Hulscher JB, van Sandick JW, Tijssen JG, Obertop H, van Lanschot JJ (2000) The recurrence pattern of esophageal carcinoma after transhiatal resection. J Am Coll Surg 191:143–148
14. Hulscher JB, van Sandick JW, de Boer AG, Wijnhoven BP, Tijssen JG, Fockens P et al (2002) Extended transthoracic resection compared with limited transhiatal resection for adenocarcinoma of the esophagus. N Engl J Med 347:1662–1669
15. Omloo JM, Lagarde SM, Hulscher JB, Reitsma JB, Fockens P, van Dekken H et al (2007) Extended transthoracic resection compared with limited transhiatal resection for adenocarcinoma of the mid/distal esophagus: five-year survival of a randomized clinical trial. Ann Surg 246:992–1000
16. Dresner SM, Griffin SM (2000) Pattern of recurrence following radical oesophagectomy with two-field lymphadenectomy. Br J Surg 87:1426–1433

17. Hagen JA, DeMeester SR, Peters JH, Chandrasoma P, DeMeester TR (2001) Curative resection for esophageal adenocarcinoma: analysis of 100 en bloc esophagectomies. Ann Surg 234:520–530
18. Goldminc M, Maddern G, Le Prise E, Meunier B, Campion JP, Launois B (1993) Oesophagectomy by a transhiatal approach or thoracotomy: a prospective randomized trial. Br J Surg 80:367–370
19. Chu KM, Law SY, Fok M, Wong J (1997) A prospective randomized comparison of transhiatal and transthoracic resection for lower-third esophageal carcinoma. Am J Surg 174:320–324
20. Omloo JM, Law SY, Launois B, Le Prise E, Wong J, van Berge Henegouwen MI et al (2009) Short and long-term advantages of transhiatal and transthoracic oesophageal cancer resection. Eur J Surg Oncol 35: 793–797
21. Peyre CG, Hagen JA, DeMeester SR, Van Lanschot JJ, Holscher A, Griffin SM et al (2008) Predicting systemic disease in patients with esophageal cancer after esophagectomy: a multinational study on the significance of the number of involved lymph nodes. Ann Surg 248:979–985
22. Peyre CG, Hagen JA, DeMeester SR, Altorki NK, Ancona E, Griffin SM et al (2008) The number of lymph nodes removed predicts survival in esophageal cancer: an international study on the impact of extent of surgical resection. Ann Surg 248:549–556
23. Rizk NP, Ishwaran H, Rice TW, Chen LQ, Schipper PH, Kesler KA et al (2010) Optimum lymphadenectomy for esophageal cancer. Ann Surg 251:46–50
24. Groth SS, Virnig BA, Whitson BA, DeFor TE, Li ZZ, Tuttle TM et al (2010) Determination of the minimum number of lymph nodes to examine to maximize survival in patients with esophageal carcinoma: data from the Surveillance Epidemiology and End Results database. J Thorac Cardiovasc Surg 139:612–620
25. Altorki NK, Zhou XK, Stiles B, Port JL, Paul S, Lee PC et al (2008) Total number of resected lymph nodes predicts survival in esophageal cancer. Ann Surg 248:221–226
26. Lerut T, De Leyn P, Coosemans W, Van Raemdonck D, Scheys I, LeSaffre E (1992) Surgical strategies in esophageal carcinoma with emphasis on radical lymphadenectomy. Ann Surg 216:583–590
27. Junginger T, Gockel I, Heckhoff S (2006) A comparison of transhiatal and transthoracic resections on the prognosis in patients with squamous cell carcinoma of the esophagus. Eur J Surg Oncol 32:749–755
28. Horstmann O, Verreet PR, Becker H, Ohmann C, Roher HD (1995) Transhiatal oesophagectomy compared with transthoracic resection and systematic lymphadenectomy for the treatment of oesophageal cancer. Eur J Surg 161:557–567
29. Morgan MA, Lewis WG, Hopper AN, Escofet X, Havard TJ, Brewster AE et al (2007) Prospective comparison of transthoracic versus transhiatal esophagectomy following neoadjuvant therapy for esophageal cancer. Dis Esophagus 20:225–231
30. Kato H, Watanabe H, Tachimori Y, Iizuka T (1991) Evaluation of neck lymph node dissection for thoracic esophageal carcinoma. Ann Thorac Surg 51:931–935
31. Altorki NK, Skinner DB (1997) Occult cervical nodal metastasis in esophageal cancer: preliminary results of three-field lymphadenectomy. J Thorac Cardiovasc Surg 113:540–544
32. Griffin SM, Burt AD, Jennings NA (2011) Lymph node metastasis in early esophageal adenocarcinoma. Ann Surg 254:731–736
33. Barbour AP, Jones M, Brown I, Gotley DC, Martin I, Thomas J et al (2010) Risk stratification for early esophageal adenocarcinoma: analysis of lymphatic spread and prognostic factors. Ann Surg Oncol 17: 2494–2502
34. Stein HJ, Hutter J, Feith M, von Rahden BH (2007) Limited surgical resection and jejunal interposition for early adenocarcinoma of the distal esophagus. Semin Thorac Cardiovasc Surg 19:72–78
35. Lamb PJ, Griffin SM, Burt AD, Lloyd J, Karat D, Hayes N (2005) Sentinel node biopsy to evaluate the metastatic dissemination of oesophageal adenocarcinoma. Br J Surg 92:60–67

Definitive Chemoradiation Therapy 11

Joel Shapiro and J. Jan B. van Lanschot

11.1 Introduction

Treatment of esophageal cancer has become increasingly complex over the last three decades. Historically, both primary surgery and primary radiotherapy have been used to treat locally advanced esophageal cancer. These surgical and nonsurgical treatment approaches developed independently into acceptable treatment options [1–5] and both improved over time due to advances in pre-treatment staging [6–8] and either improved surgical [9–11] or radiation techniques [12, 13], respectively. However, due to a lack in high-quality randomized controlled data, clinical opinions and institutional preferences still dominate treatment selection.

In this chapter we intend to give an overview of the historical progression of the nonsurgical treatment paradigm for potentially curative esophageal cancer.

J. Shapiro • J.J.B. van Lanschot (✉)
Department of Surgery, Erasmus Medical Center, Dr. Molewaterplein 50, Rotterdam, Zuid-Holland 3015 GE, The Netherlands
e-mail: j.vanlanschot@erasmusmc.nl

11.2 Overview of Treatment Paradigms

Before the 1980s, well over 95 % of all diagnosed esophageal cancers were considered to be of squamous origin [1, 14]. Squamous cell carcinomas of the esophagus were then treated by either primary surgical resection or by primary radiotherapy alone [1, 2].

In their seminal reviews Earlam and Cunha-Melo gave an extensive overview of the published literature on treatment outcomes for primary surgery and primary radiotherapy for squamous cell carcinomas of the esophagus [1, 2]. The only treatment option then for adenocarcinomas of the esophagus that was considered curative was primary surgical resection [1]. The results were sobering: 1- and 5-year survival rates after surgical resection were 18 and 4 %, respectively. Survival rates after primary radiotherapy were similarly disappointing: 18 and 6 %, respectively.

Although survival seemed similar after either treatment option, a strong negative patient selection bias was present in the primary radiotherapy data. Patients who underwent primary radiotherapy had most likely been rejected for surgical resection because of extensive disease or because of severe comorbidities. These negative selection criteria possibly masked a more favorable outcome after radiotherapy. If patient selection had been more similar between the two treatment

L. Bonavina (ed.), *Innovation in Esophageal Surgery*,
DOI 10.1007/978-88-470-2469-4_11, © Springer-Verlag Italia 2012

paradigms, primary radiotherapy might have resulted in superior survival rates.

These results indicate that at that time primary radiotherapy should have been considered at least as effective as primary surgery in the treatment of potentially curative squamous cell carcinoma of the esophagus.

11.3 Addition of Chemotherapy to Primary Radiotherapy

Chemotherapy and radiotherapy interact in several ways. One mode of interaction is that they both target different tumor cell populations within the primary tumor ('additive effect'). Chemotherapy may also be effective against micrometastases, while radiotherapy is active only locoregionally ('spatial cooperation'). Chemotherapy also has an added local effect by increasing the sensitivity of cells to radiotherapy ('synergistic effect'). Mechanisms of increased sensitivity to radiotherapy include: (1) synchronizing cells to a specific cell-cycle phase, (2) decreased repopulation after individual radiotherapy fractions and (3) enhanced tissue reoxygenation, due to tumor shrinkage [15–17].

11.4 Sequential Chemoradiotherapy

A Cochrane meta-analysis from 2006 by Wong and Malthaner [18] reviewed the reported effects of sequential chemoradiotherapy on overall survival as compared to radiotherapy alone. This meta-analysis was based on 857 patients from eight included studies [19–26] and concluded that sequential chemoradiotherapy did not improve outcome as compared to primary radiotherapy alone (mortality hazard ratio (HR) 0.87, 95 % confidence interval (CI) 0.74–1.02).

11.5 Concurrent Chemoradiotherapy

The Radiation Therapy Oncology Group (RTOG) performed a phase III trial (RTOG 85-01) [27] comparing concurrent chemoradiotherapy to radiotherapy alone for *potentially curable* esophageal cancer (both squamous cell- and adenocarcinoma). The chemoradiation regimen consisted of two concurrent courses of 5-fluorouracil and cisplatin with 50 Gy radiotherapy followed by two additional courses of the same chemotherapy regimen. The radiotherapy-alone regimen consisted of 64 Gy given in 32 fractions. On interim analysis a significant survival difference in favor of the chemoradiotherapy arm (median survival 12.5 versus 8.9 months respectively, $p<0.001$) was found, which led to an early closure of the trial. Treatment related toxicity was increased in the chemoradiotherapy arm compared to the radiotherapy alone arm (severe toxicity: 44 versus 25 %, life-threatening toxicity: 20 versus 3 %, respectively). Late toxicity was not increased as has been reported in other studies with concomitant chemoradiotherapy [28]. al-Sarraf et al. [29] reported on an additional group of patients treated with the same chemoradiotherapy regimen. The survival of this non-randomized group was identical to that of the randomized group of patients. The long-term results of the RTOG 85-01 trial were published by Cooper et al. [30] in 1999. These results showed significantly improved 5-year overall survival rates for patients treated with chemoradiotherapy as compared to radiotherapy alone (26 %, 95 % CI (15–37 %) and 0 %, respectively).

In the subsequent RTOG 94–05 trial (USA Intergroup 123) [31] patients were randomized to either receive the standard chemoradiotherapy regimen (50 Gy), as was used in the RTOG 85-01 trial, or the same chemotherapy regimen combined with a higher radiotherapy dose (64.8 Gy). After an interim analysis this trial was closed prematurely because of a high number of treatment-related deaths in the high-dose radiotherapy arm. There was no significant difference in median or 2-year survival between the two arms. Prior to this study the Intergroup had performed a phase II study (INT 0122) [31]. In this study the radiotherapy dose was increased from 50 to 64.8 Gy, the number of chemotherapy courses from 4 to 5 and 5-fluorouracil was given for 5 days instead of 4. Four of the 45 entered patients (9 %) died due to treatment-related toxicity.

The European Organization for Research and Treatment of Cancer (EORTC) reported on a randomized study of split-course radiotherapy (2 × 20 Gy, 4 Gy each fraction, 5 fractions per week with a 2 week gap) with or without two courses of cisplatin 100 mg/m^2 given 3 or 4 days before the start of radiotherapy and four courses afterwards [25]. The median overall survival was not significantly different between the two groups (7.9 and 9.6 months for patients in the radiotherapy- and chemoradiotherapy arm, respectively). This split course radiotherapy and timing of chemotherapy are considered suboptimal nowadays.

The same Cochrane meta-analysis by Wong and Malthaner [18] reviewed the reported effects of concurrent chemoradiotherapy on overall survival as compared to radiotherapy alone, including the data from the RTOG 85-01 trial. The meta-analysis was based on 998 patients from 11 included studies [30, 32–41] and concluded that concurrent chemoradiotherapy did improve overall survival significantly as compared to primary radiotherapy alone (mortality (HR) 0.73, 95 % CI 0.74–1.02).

These studies and meta-analysis show that concurrent chemoradiotherapy is recommended over radiotherapy alone as a non-surgical therapy for potentially curable esophageal cancer. A higher dose of radiotherapy (64 versus 50 Gy) in combination with chemotherapy increases toxicity rates without an advantage in survival.

11.6 Definitive Chemoradiotherapy Versus Neoadjuvant Chemoradiotherapy Plus Surgery

In recent years two randomized controlled trials have been reported in the literature comparing definitive chemoradiotherapy (dCRT) to neoadjuvant chemoradiotherapy plus surgery (nCRT+S) for squamous cell carcinoma of the esophagus.

The first study by Stahl et al. [42] included 172 patients between 1994 and 2002 from 11 German centers. It compared definitive chemoradiotherapy (without salvage surgery) with neoadjuvant chemoradiotherapy plus surgery for

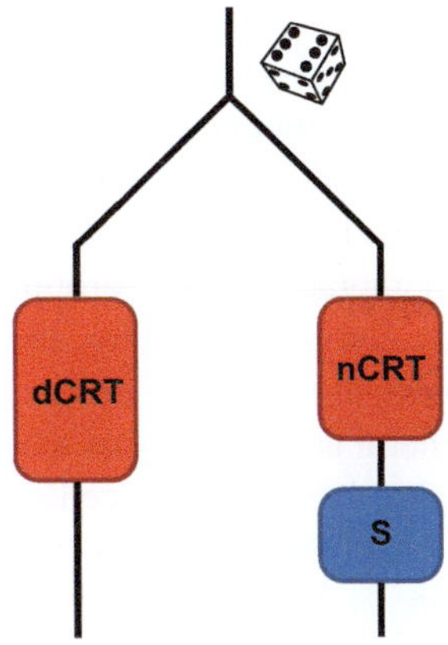

Fig. 11.1 Treatment design of the study by Stahl et al. [42]. *dCRT* definitive chemoradiation therapy, *nCRT* neoadjuvant chemoradiation therapy, *S* surgery. Only esophageal squamous cell tumors were included. *Dice* represents moment of randomization

'locally advanced' (i.e. T3-4, N0-1, M0) esophageal squamous cell carcinomas (Fig. 11.1). Patients with adenocarcinomas were not included. The trial was powered to show *equivalence* within a range of 15 % with overall survival as the primary endpoint. After induction chemotherapy with cisplatin, 5-fluorouracil, etoposide and leucovorin patients were randomized to either receive definitive concurrent chemoradiotherapy with cisplatin, etoposide and 60–65 Gy of radiation or to receive concurrent chemoradiotherapy with cisplatin, etoposide and 40 Gy of radiation, followed by transthoracic esophagectomy. Patients were staged with endoscopic ultrasonography (EUS) and computed tomography (CT) and stratified by center, tumor- and node stage, completeness of EUS, sex and extent of weight loss in 2 months prior to diagnosis. Two-year survival was 35.4 % in the definitive chemoradiotherapy arm and 39.9 % in the neoadjuvant chemoradiotherapy plus surgery arm (p=0.007, i.e. the chance that there is a true difference of more than 15 %). Freedom from local progression was worse in the definitive chemoradiotherapy group as compared to the neoadjuvant chemoradiotherapy plus surgery group (40.7 vs. 64.3 % respectively; HR 2.1 p=.003). A significant difference was found in treatment related mortality: 3.5 % in the definitive chemoradiotherapy arm and 12.8 % in the neoadjuvant chemoradiotherapy plus surgery arm (χ^2, p=.03). In summary, there was no difference in overall survival; however local failure was more common, and treatment-related death less common in the definitive chemoradiotherapy group.

Although commendable for its complexity, several aspects of this trial's design and analysis limit the general applicability of these results.

First, only 'locally advanced' tumors were included (T3, T4). This allows only limited extrapolation to less advanced tumors (≤T2). Second, the groups of patients were small for an equivalence design, as is reflected by the uncommonly broad equivalence range of 15 %. Choosing a $\delta = -0.15$ allows for a difference in overall survival of up to 15 % to be considered equivalent. This is too broad, as it surpasses the survival differences considered clinically relevant in most superiority designs [43]. From a patient's perspective: is an individual patient willing to accept a potential decrease in long term survival of up to 15 % by refraining from surgical resection? In general, in contrast to superiority studies, equivalence or non-inferiority trials should be analyzed by both *per protocol* and *intention to treat* analyses, not just by *intention to treat* as was done in the Stahl et al. paper. Including protocol violators and withdrawals as is done in an *intention to treat* analysis will increase the blurring between two treatment groups and thus increases the chance of falsely finding equivalence or non-inferiority [43]. This is especially relevant, since 29 of 86 patients randomized to neoadjuvant chemoradiotherapy plus surgery arm did not actually undergo surgery.

Third, the reported in-hospital mortality rate and the overall treatment-related mortality rate in the neoadjuvant chemoradiotherapy plus surgery arm (86 patients) were 11.3 and 12.8 % respectively. This is high compared to large series in high volume centers and might have biased the results in favor of equivalence. As mentioned above, 29 of 86 patients randomized to the neoadjuvant chemoradiotherapy plus surgery arm did not actually undergo surgery. If one recalculates the overall treatment-related mortality for those patients that actually received surgery, the rate increases to 19.3 %. It should be noted that this rate greatly exceeds the commonly reported mortality rates for this type of surgery [9, 10, 13, 21]. For comparison, in the recent CROSS trial, the in-hospital mortality rate of the neoadjuvant chemoradiotherapy plus surgery was 3.8 % [44].

In 2008, Stahl et al. reported their long-term results [45], showing 5- and 10-year overall survival rates of 17.0 and 12.2 % respectively in the definitive chemoradiotherapy group and 27.9 and 19.2 % in the neoadjuvant chemoradiotherapy plus surgery group. When adjusted for disease-specific survival, the 10-year survival becomes 12.2 % for the definitive chemoradiotherapy group versus 24.8 % for the neoadjuvant chemoradiotherapy plus surgery group. Although these results fall within their chosen limit of equivalence, these data show an overall survival difference of 11 % at 5 years, and a disease-specific survival difference of 12.6 % at 10 years, which is a survival reduction of more than 50 %.

In conclusion, the Stahl et al. [42, 45] study has addressed an important topic that is currently under debate – definitive chemoradiotherapy as an alternative to neoadjuvant chemoradiotherapy plus surgery in esophageal squamous cell carcinoma – and demonstrates the complexity of conducting randomized controlled trials in the field of multimodality treatment for squamous cell carcinomas of the esophagus, especially when comparing surgical and non-surgical treatment arms.

However, we feel the study has two major drawbacks. It is underpowered, making it difficult to draw reliable conclusions from the data and local failure was more common in the definitive chemoradiotherapy group. This leaves room, in our view, for future trials which are adequately powered and incorporate a more effective neoadjuvant regimen to decrease local failure rates.

The second randomized controlled trial (FFCD 9102) was reported by Bedenne et al. in 2007 [46]. This French study used an equivalence design to compare definitive chemoradiotherapy (dCRT) with neoadjuvant chemoradiotherapy plus surgery (nCRT+S) (Fig. 11.2). Inclusion criteria were resectable T3N0-1M0 squamous cell- or adenocarcinomas

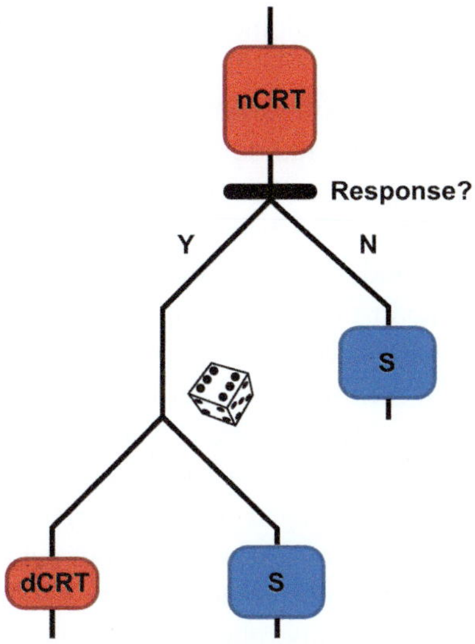

Fig. 11.2 Treatment design of the study by Bedenne et al. [46]. *dCRT* definitive chemoradiation therapy, *nCRT* neoadjuvant chemoradiation therapy, *S* surgery, *US* ultrasonography. Both squamous cell- and adenocarcinomas were included. Clinical response was evaluated by esophagography, abdominal US, chest X-ray and if possible endoscopic US. *Dice* represents moment of randomization

of the esophagus (squamous cell carcinomas >90 %) in patients eligible to undergo surgery and chemoradiotherapy. Staging was done by CT. All patients were treated with two cycles of fluorouracil and cisplatin combined with one of two possible schedules of radiotherapy: 30 Gy in two split courses or 46 Gy given continuously. Only patients who had an objective clinical response or an improvement of dysphagia after neoadjuvant chemoradiotherapy were randomized (259/444, 58.3 %). Clinical response was evaluated by esophagography, abdominal ultrasonography, chest X-ray and if possible endoscopic ultrasonography. Both sequential- and concurrent chemoradiotherapy were used in both definitive- and neoadjuvant chemoradiotherapy regimens. The primary endpoint was overall survival and secondary endpoints were duration of hospital stay, quality of life, type of recurrence, and procedures for dysphagia. Treatment was considered equivalent if the difference in 2-year survival rates between the two treatment arms was less than 10 %.

Two-year survival rates for the definitive chemoradiotherapy arm and neoadjuvant chemoradiotherapy plus surgery arm were 39.8 and 33.6 % respectively, leading to the conclusion that the difference in survival between the two treatment arms was less than 10 % and thus equivalent ($p=0.03$, i.e. the chance that there is an actual difference of more than 10 %). Secondary endpoints included 3-month mortality (0.8 versus 9.3 %, $p=0.0003$) and length of hospital stay (52 versus 68 days, $p=0.015$), which both favored the definitive chemoradiotherapy arm, whereas locoregional relapse (43.0 versus 33.6 %, HR 1.63, $p=0.03$) and treatment for dysphagia (46 versus 24 %, $p=0.001$) both favored the neoadjuvant chemoradiotherapy plus surgery arm. Although locoregional recurrence was lower in the neoadjuvant chemoradiotherapy plus surgery group, it did not have an impact on survival, as evidenced by the equivalence of median- and 2-year survival between the two treatment groups.

In 2008, Jouve et al. [47] published survival data on the *non-randomized* patients of the FFCD 9102 trial. Non-randomized patients that were operated on had improved median overall survival as compared to non-randomized non-operated patients: 17.3 and 6.1 months, respectively ($p<0.0001$). Moreover, non-randomized patients that were operated on did not differ in their median overall survival compared to the randomized patients: 17.3 and 18.9 months, respectively ($p<0.58$).

General applicability of the conclusions from the FFCD 9102 trial is limited by a few remarkable results. First, the reported survival rates seem to differ substantially from the 2-year survival rates reported elsewhere, e.g. the CROSS trial [44] which reported 2-year survival rates of 67 and 52 % in the neoadjuvant plus surgery group and surgery alone group, respectively. Even when considering the less advanced 'average' disease stage of the CROSS patients, we find the difference in survival between the CROSS and FFCD 9102 trials striking. Possible explanations why the FFCD 9102 trial has lower survival rates could be the understaging of disease due to a lack of regular EUS as part of the standard diagnostic work-up. Neither of the two arms represents the accepted golden standard. This means that equivalence could also be found between two arms when the true superior arm underperforms. Therefore, the found equivalence between the definitive chemoradiotherapy and neoadjuvant chemoradiotherapy plus surgery arms could also be attributed to a lower than expected overall survival rate for the neoadjuvant chemoradiotherapy plus surgery arm, as compared to other recent multimodality treatment trials. This point holds true for the Stahl et al. trial [42, 45] as well. Second, the chemoradiotherapy regimen in the FFCD 9102 trial seems to result in less R0 resections as compared, for example, to the CROSS trial: 75 versus 92.3 %, respectively.

The last striking result is the significant difference in freedom from locoregional progression: 64.3 and 40.7 % (p=0.003) for the definitive chemoradiotherapy and neoadjuvant chemoradiotherapy plus surgery arms, respectively. It is hard to imagine that differences in locoregional recurrence after definitive chemoradiotherapy or neoadjuvant chemoradiotherapy plus surgery would not strongly correlate with eventual differences in overall survival. Most likely the length of follow-up as reported in this paper was too short to reflect survival differences. It is conceivable that a difference of more than 20 % in freedom from locoregional progression in favor of neoadjuvant chemoradiotherapy plus surgery might very well cause this trial to become non-equivalent at longer follow-up.

In summary, we believe that an important question remains unanswered. Namely, is there a role for definitive chemoradiotherapy in selected patients with esophageal squamous cell carcinoma, and perhaps even esophageal adenocarcinoma?

11.7 Addition of Salvage Surgery to Definitive Chemoradiotherapy

More recently, several high volume centers have reported their – mostly retrospective – results of patients treated by salvage esophagectomy for residual or recurrent locoregional disease after definitive chemoradiotherapy with curative intent [48–59].

The concept of salvage surgery after failed definitive chemoradiotherapy became viable thanks to two important developments. The first development was a sharp decline in perioperative morbidity and mortality for esophageal resections in the last decades [60]. This is due in part to better patient selection [61, 62], improvements in surgical technique and perioperative management [11, 63–65] and centralization of care [66, 67]. This decline in surgery-associated morbidity and mortality made delayed surgical resection a more attractive salvage option in those patients in whom definitive chemoradiotherapy had failed.

The second important development was the addition of neoadjuvant chemoradiotherapy regimens to primary surgical treatment for esophageal cancer [44, 68–70]. This development familiarized surgeons with the resection of an irradiated esophagus and showed the feasibility of performing an esophagectomy at extended time intervals after completion of neoadjuvant chemoradiotherapy, without significant increases in morbidity and/or mortality [71, 72].

The overall decline in surgery-associated morbidity and mortality, together with an accumulating experience in esophageal resections after neoadjuvant chemoradiotherapy allowed for salvage surgery after definitive chemoradiotherapy to be undertaken at an acceptable risk [46–57] .

A recent non-randomized phase II trial by Swisher et al. [73] examined the 1-year survival benefit of adding salvage surgery to definitive chemoradiotherapy. Definitive chemoradiotherapy consisted of two cycles of induction chemotherapy with 5-fluorouracil (5-FU), cisplatin and paclitaxel, followed by concurrent chemoradiotherapy with 50.4 Gy and 5-FU with cisplatin. Following completion of chemoradiotherapy, patients were assessed for residual cancer with esophagogastroduodenoscopy (EGD), and EUS and CT scans of the chest and abdomen. A positron emission tomography (PET) scan was optional but strongly recommended. Histological proof of residual or recurrent locoregional disease was not absolutely required to consider patients for salvage surgery. If there was no clinical suspicion of residual cancer, patients were followed closely with serial EGD, EUS and CT scans of the chest and abdomen. Again, PET scans were optional but strongly recommended.

For this study, 18 medical centers enrolled 43 patients of whom 41 were eligible for analysis. Both squamous cell carcinomas and adenocarcinomas were included: 11 (27 %) and 30 (73 %) respectively. Of these 41 patients 21 patients (51 %) underwent salvage surgery. Seventeen patients underwent salvage surgery because of suspicion of residual disease, 3 patients because of suspicion of recurrent disease and 1 patient at his own request. All resected patients, except for the single patient who requested surgical resection without any clinical suspicion of cancer, had tumor cells present in the resected specimen. Median follow-up time was 16.1 months and estimated 1-year overall survival was 71 % (95 % CI 54–82 %). Because 1-year overall survival did not reach the preset level of 77.5 %, these results were not considered promising enough to be tested in a phase III trial.

This trial is the first prospective investigation of the value of salvage surgery after unsuccessful definitive chemoradiotherapy for esophageal cancer. Unfortunately overall 1 year survival did not reach the trial's 1-year survival rate target (71 % instead of 77.5 %). However, a few comments can be made on this. First, the target 1-year survival rate, 77.5 %, falls within the trial's estimated 1-year overall survival 95 % confidence interval (54–82 %), meaning that the true 1-year overall survival rate might actually be much closer to the target 1-year survival rate than was assumed in the discussion of this study.

Second, as the authors already mentioned, the target 1-year survival rate of 77.5 % was determined from the Radiation Therapy Oncology Group (RTOG) database, which consists of mainly squamous cell carcinoma patients, possibly negatively biasing current patient populations, which consist of a majority of adenocarcinoma patients. Third, 3 of 41 patients (7.3 %) died due to chemoradiotherapy-related causes. If these deaths could have been prevented, perhaps by taking out the induction chemotherapy from the treatment regimen, the target 1-year survival rate might then have been achieved.

Taken together these considerations point towards a more positive conclusion from this trial than perhaps was made by its authors.

11.8 Future Perspectives

Treatment for esophageal cancer has evolved in recent decades. It is now clear that when esophageal cancer is treated non-surgically, definitive concurrent chemoradiotherapy is the preferred treatment. However, what still remains unclear is whether the addition of surgery – as a standard or as a salvage procedure – has any benefit for long-term overall survival in 'definitive' chemoradiotherapy.

Ever since the addition of chemotherapy and selective salvage surgery to primary radiotherapy and the addition of neoadjuvant chemoradiotherapy to primary surgery, both the non-surgical and the surgical treatment paradigms have moved closer towards each other (Fig. 11.3). In fact, it may be debated whether there is any essential difference left. Perhaps the next trial should not focus on the addition of salvage surgery to a definitive chemoradiotherapy regimen, but rather focus on applying 'planned' surgery more selectively. A mild, yet effective neoadjuvant regimen, as was used in the CROSS trial [44], caused relatively low morbidity and mortality while achieving 49 and 23 % pathologically complete responses in squamous cell carcinomas and adenocarcinomas, respectively. These results indicate that the neoadjuvant regimen used in the CROSS trial was as effective as most definitive chemoradiotherapy regimens while being very well tolerated by patients.

Therefore, we are currently designing a new trial in The Netherlands that will compare the neoadjuvant chemoradiotherapy plus surgery arm from the CROSS trial with a neoadjuvant chemoradiotherapy plus 'surgery as needed' arm, in which surgery will be offered only to those patients who have signs of residual or recurrent disease without any signs of distant dissemination. The main objective of this new trial will be

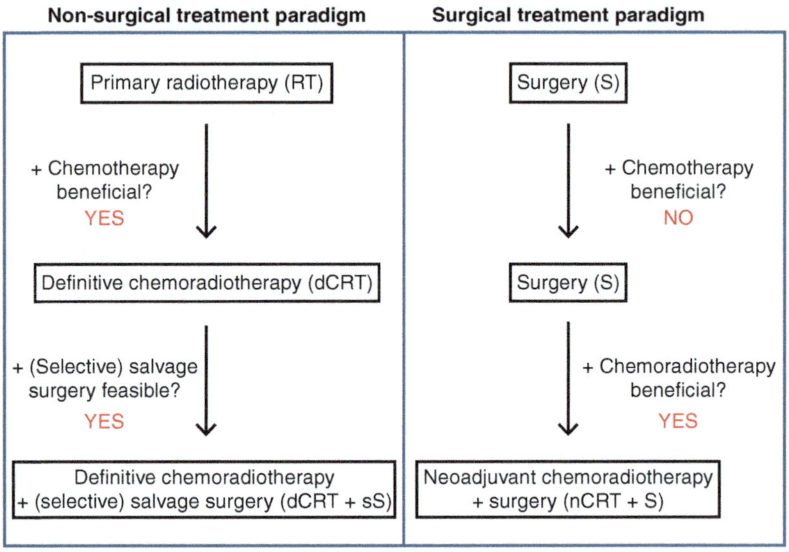

Fig. 11.3 Historical progression of both treatment paradigms

to assess whether for patients with either squamous cell- or adenocarcinoma of the esophagus we can improve upon our results from the CROSS trial by achieving similar overall-survival results with less patients being exposed to surgery after neoadjuvant chemoradiotherapy.

Key Points

- Overall 5-year survival rates after potentially curative esophagectomy have improved but rarely exceed 40 %
- Neoadjuvant chemoradiation therapy plus surgery has the potential to increase R0 resection rate and pathological CR rate in both adenocarcinoma and squamous-cell carcinoma
- The role for definitive chemoradiation therapy is still highly debated
- Phase III studies on salvage esophagectomy for residual or recurrent disease after definitive chemoradiation therapy with curative intent are lacking
- The new CROSS trial has been designed as a definitive treatment until the patient shows a locoregional recurrence without signs of disseminated disease

References

1. Earlam R, Cunha-Melo JR (1980) Oesophageal squamous cell carcinoma: I. A critical review of surgery. Br J Surg 67:381–390
2. Earlam R, Cunha-Melo JR (1980) Oesophogeal squamous cell carcinoms: II. A critical view of radiotherapy. Br J Surg 67:457–461
3. Hancock SL, Glatstein E (1984) Radiation therapy of esophageal cancer. Semin Oncol 11:144–158
4. Mahoney JL, Condon RE (1987) Adenocarcinoma of the esophagus. Ann Surg 205:557–562
5. Sykes AJ et al (1998) Radical radiotherapy for carcinoma of the oesophagus: an effective alternative to surgery. Radiother Oncol 48(1):15–21
6. Lightdale CJ (1992) Endoscopic ultrasonography in the diagnosis, staging and follow-up of esophageal and gastric cancer. Endoscopy 24(Suppl 1): 297–303
7. Block MI et al (1997) Improvement in staging of esophageal cancer with the addition of positron emission tomography. Ann Thorac Surg 64(3):770–776
8. Hulscher JB et al (2000) Laparoscopy and laparoscopic ultrasonography in staging carcinoma of the gastric cardia. Eur J Surg 166(11):862–865
9. Skinner DB et al (1986) Selection of operation for esophageal cancer based on staging. Ann Surg 204(4): 391–401
10. Van Lanschot JJ et al (1999) Randomized comparison of prevertebral and retrosternal gastric tube reconstruction after resection of oesophageal carcinoma. Br J Surg 86(1):102–108
11. Hulscher JBF et al (2002) Extended transthoracic resection compared with limited transhiatal resection for adenocarcinoma of the esophagus. N Engl J Med 347(21):1662–1669

12. Gaspar LE et al (1997) A phase I/II study of external beam radiation, brachytherapy and concurrent chemotherapy in localized cancer of the esophagus (RTOG 92-07): preliminary toxicity report. Int J Radiat Oncol Biol Phys 37(3):593–599
13. Toita T et al (2001) Concurrent chemoradiotherapy for squamous cell carcinoma of thoracic esophagus: feasibility and outcome of large regional field and high-dose external beam boost irradiation. Jpn J Clin Oncol 31(8):375–381
14. Raphael HA, Ellis FH Jr, Dockerty MB (1966) Primary adenocarcinoma of the esophagus: 18-year review and review of literature. Ann Surg 164(5):785–796
15. Tannock IF (1996) Treatment of cancer with radiation and drugs. J Clin Oncol 14(12):3156–3174
16. Hennequin C, Favaudon V (2002) Biological basis for chemo-radiotherapy interactions. Eur J Cancer 38(2): 223–230
17. Choy H, Kim DW (2003) Chemotherapy and irradiation interaction. Semin Oncol 30(Supplement 9(0)): 3–10
18. Wong R, Malthaner R (2006) Combined chemotherapy and radiotherapy (without surgery) compared with radiotherapy alone in localized carcinoma of the esophagus. Cochrane Database Syst Rev (1): CD002092
19. Roussel A et al (1989) Palliative therapy of inoperable oesophageal carcinoma with radiotherapy and methotrexate: final results of a controlled clinical trial. Int J Radiat Oncol Biol Phys 16(1):67–72
20. Hishikawa Y, Miura T, Oshitani T, Yoshimura H, Ono K, Takahashi M et al (1991) A randomized prospective study of adjuvant chemotherapy after radiotherapy in unresectable esophageal carcinoma. Dis Esophagus 4(2):85–90
21. Zhou JC (1991) Randomized trial of combined chemotherapy including high dose cisplatin and radiotherapy for esophageal cancer. Zhonghua Zhong Liu Za Zhi 13(4):291–294
22. Hatlevoll R et al (1992) Bleomycin/cis-platin as neoadjuvant chemotherapy before radical radiotherapy in localized, inoperable carcinoma of the esophagus. A prospective randomized multicentre study: the second Scandinavian trial in esophageal cancer. Radiother Oncol 24(2):114–116
23. Lu XJ, Miao RH, Li XQ (1995) Combination of selective arterial infusion chemotherapy with radiotherapy in the treatment of advanced esophageal carcinoma. Chin J Clin Oncol 22(4):262–265
24. Tian DL (2000) Random study in radiotherapy and combined chemotherapy for advanced esophageal carcinoma of 112 patients. Chin Clin Med 7(4):409–410
25. Wobbes T et al (2001) Prospective randomised study of split-course radiotherapy versus cisplatin plus split-course radiotherapy in inoperable squamous cell carcinoma of the oesophagus. Eur J Cancer 37(4):470–477
26. Ji B et al (2002) Prospective randomized study on inductive chemotherapy plus radiotherapy for patients with upper and middle esophageal carcinoma. Chin J Radiat Oncol 11(1):12–14
27. Herskovic A et al (1992) Combined chemotherapy and radiotherapy compared with radiotherapy alone in patients with cancer of the esophagus. N Engl J Med 326(24):1593–1598
28. Schaake-Koning C et al (1992) Effects of concomitant cisplatin and radiotherapy on inoperable non-small-cell lung cancer. N Engl J Med 326(8):524–530
29. al-Sarraf M et al (1997) Progress report of combined chemoradiotherapy versus radiotherapy alone in patients with esophageal cancer: an intergroup study. J Clin Oncol 15(1):277–284
30. Cooper JS et al (1999) Chemoradiotherapy of locally advanced esophageal cancer: long-term follow-up of a prospective randomized trial (RTOG 85-01). Radiation Therapy Oncology Group. JAMA 281(17):1623–1627
31. Minsky BD et al (2002) INT 0123 (Radiation Therapy Oncology Group 94-05) phase III trial of combined-modality therapy for esophageal cancer: high-dose versus standard-dose radiation therapy. J Clin Oncol 20(5):1167–1174
32. Earle JD et al (1980) A controlled evaluation of combined radiation and bleomycin therapy for squamous cell carcinoma of the esophagus. Int J Radiat Oncol Biol Phys 6(7):821–826
33. Andersen AP et al (1984) Irradiation, chemotherapy and surgery in esophageal cancer: a randomized clinical study. The first Scandinavian trial in esophageal cancer. Radiother Oncol 2(3):179–188
34. Zhang ZF (1984) Radiation combined with bleomycin in esophageal carcinoma – a randomized study of 99 patients. Zhonghua Zhong Liu Za Zhi 6(5):372–374
35. Araújo CMM et al (1991) A randomized trial comparing radiation therapy versus concomitant radiation therapy and chemotherapy in carcinoma of the thoracic esophagus. Cancer 67(9):2258–2261
36. Roussel A et al (1994) Results of the EORTC-GTCCT Phase III trial of irradiation vs irradiation and CDDP in inoperable esophageal cancer. In: Proceedings of annual meeting of the American Society of Clinical Oncologists, Dallas, 1994, p 199
37. Kaneta T et al (1997) Effects of combination chemoradiotherapy with daily low-dose CDDP for esophageal cancer – results of a randomized trial. Gan To Kagaku Ryoho 24(14):2099–2104
38. Slabber CF et al (1998) A randomized study of radiotherapy alone versus radiotherapy plus 5-fluorouracil and platinum in patients with inoperable, locally advanced squamous cancer of the esophagus. Am J Clin Oncol 21(5):462–465
39. Li AE et al (2000) 48 Patients with advanced esophageal cancer treated with DDP-5-FU combined radiotherapy. Chin J Clin Oncol Rehabil 7(6):79–80
40. Zhu S et al (2000) Combination of external beam and intracavitary radiation and carboplatin chemotherapy in the treatment of esophageal carcinoma. Chin J Clin Oncol 27(1):5–8
41. Gao XS et al (2002) Late course accelerated hyperfractionation radiotherapy concomitant with cisplatin in patients with esophageal carcinoma. Oncol Rep 9(4):767–772

42. Stahl M et al (2005) Chemoradiation with and without surgery in patients with locally advanced squamous cell carcinoma of the esophagus. J Clin Oncol 23(10):2310–2317
43. Piaggio G et al (2006) Reporting of noninferiority and equivalence randomized trials. JAMA 295(10): 1152–1160
44. Van der Gaast AV et al (2010) Effect of preoperative concurrent chemoradiotherapy on survival of patients with resectable esophageal or esophagogastric junction cancer: results from a multicenter randomized phase III study. ASCO annual meeting 2010. J Clin Oncol 28(15 suppl):abstr 4004
45. Stahl M et al (2008) Long-term results of a phase III study investigating chemoradiation with and without surgery in locally advanced squamous cell carcinoma (LA-SCC) of the esophagus. ASCO annual meeting. J Clin Oncol 26:(20 suppl):abstr 4530
46. Bedenne L et al (2007) Chemoradiation followed by surgery compared with chemoradiation alone in squamous cancer of the esophagus: FFCD 9102. J Clin Oncol 25(10):1160–1168
47. Jouve J et al (2008) Outcome of the nonrandomized patients in the FFCD 9102 trial: chemoradiation followed by surgery compared with chemoradiation alone in squamous cancer of the esophagus. ASCO annual meeting. J Clin Oncol 26(20 suppl):abstr 4555
48. Meunier B et al (1998) Salvage esophagectomy after unsuccessful curative chemoradiotherapy for squamous cell cancer of the esophagus. Dig Surg 15(3):224–226
49. Swisher SG et al (2002) Salvage esophagectomy for recurrent tumors after definitive chemotherapy and radiotherapy. J Thorac Cardiovasc Surg 123(1):175–183
50. Nakamura T et al (2004) Salvage esophagectomy after definitive chemotherapy and radiotherapy for advanced esophageal cancer. Am J Surg 188(3):261–266
51. Tomimaru Y et al (2006) Factors affecting the prognosis of patients with esophageal cancer undergoing salvage surgery after definitive chemoradiotherapy. J Surg Oncol 93(5):422–428
52. Oki E et al (2007) Salvage esophagectomy after definitive chemoradiotherapy for esophageal cancer. Dis Esophagus 20(4):301–304
53. Smithers BM et al (2007) Outcomes from salvage esophagectomy post definitive chemoradiotherapy compared with resection following preoperative neoadjuvant chemoradiotherapy. Dis Esophagus 20(6):471–477
54. Piessen G et al (2007) Patients with locally advanced esophageal carcinoma nonresponder to radiochemotherapy: who will benefit from surgery? Ann Surg Oncol 14(7):2036–2044
55. D'Journo XB et al (2008) Indications and outcome of salvage surgery for oesophageal cancer. Eur J Cardiothorac Surg 33(6):1117–1123
56. Borghesi S, Hawkins MA, Tait D (2008) Oesophagectomy after definitive chemoradiation in patients with locally advanced oesophageal cancer. Clin Oncol (R Coll Radiol) 20(3):221–226
57. Miyata H et al (2009) Salvage esophagectomy after definitive chemoradiotherapy for thoracic esophageal cancer. J Surg Oncol 100(6):442–446
58. Pinto CE et al (2009) Salvage esophagectomy after exclusive chemoradiotherapy: results at the Brazilian National Cancer Institute (INCA). Dis Esophagus 22(8):682–686
59. Tachimori Y et al (2009) Salvage esophagectomy after high-dose chemoradiotherapy for esophageal squamous cell carcinoma. J Thorac Cardiovasc Surg 137(1): 49–54
60. Müller JM et al (1990) Surgical therapy of oesophageal carcinoma. Br J Surg 77(8):845–857
61. Ferguson MK, Durkin AE (2002) Preoperative prediction of the risk of pulmonary complications after esophagectomy for cancer. J Thorac Cardiovasc Surg 123(4):661–669
62. Grotenhuis BA et al (2010) Preoperative risk assessment and prevention of complications in patients with esophageal cancer. J Surg Oncol 101(3):270–278
63. Law S, Wong J (2005) Current management of esophageal cancer. J Gastrointest Surg 9(2):291–310
64. Omloo JMT et al (2007) Extended transthoracic resection compared with limited transhiatal resection for adenocarcinoma of the mid/distal esophagus: five-year survival of a randomized clinical trial. Ann Surg 246(6): 992–1001
65. Ju-Mei N (2008) Perioperative anesthetic management for esophagectomy. Anesthesiol Clin 26(2):293–304
66. Verhoef C et al (2007) Better survival in patients with esophageal cancer after surgical treatment in university hospitals: a plea for performance by surgical oncologists. Ann Surg Oncol 14(5):1678–1687
67. Wouters MW et al (2008) High-volume versus low-volume for esophageal resections for cancer: the essential role of case-mix adjustments based on clinical data. Ann Surg Oncol 15(1):80–87
68. Thirion PG et al (2007) Individual patient data-based meta-analysis assessing pre-operative chemotherapy in resectable oesophageal carcinoma. ASCO meeting abstracts. J Clin Oncol 25(18 suppl):abstr 4512
69. Thirion P, Maillard E, Pignon J (2008) Individual patient data-based meta-analysis assessing the effect of preoperative chemo-radiotherapy in resectable oesophageal carcinoma. Int J Radiat Oncol Biol Phys 72(1):S71–S72
70. Sjoquist KM et al (2011) Survival after neoadjuvant chemotherapy or chemoradiotherapy for resectable oesophageal carcinoma: an updated meta-analysis. Lancet Oncol 12(7):681–692
71. Ruol A et al (2010) Interval between neoadjuvant chemoradiotherapy and surgery for squamous cell carcinoma of the thoracic esophagus: does delayed surgery have an impact on outcome? Ann Surg 252(5):788–796
72. Kim JY et al (2012) Does the timing of esophagectomy after chemoradiation affect outcome? Ann Thorac Surg 93(1):207–212; discussion 212–213. Epub 2011 Oct 1
73. Swisher SG et al (2012) A phase II study of a paclitaxel-based chemoradiation regimen with selective surgical salvage for resectable locoregionally advanced esophageal cancer: initial reporting of RTOG 0246. Int J Radiat Oncol Biol Phys 82(5):1967–1972, Epub 2011 Apr 18

The Art and Science of Esophageal Anastomosis

12

Simon Law

12.1 Introduction

The esophageal anastomosis remains a controversial subject. Its importance lies in its propensity to leak, develop stricture, and tumor recurrence at the anastomosis after esophagectomy for cancer defeats one of the main objectives of the surgery: the relief of dysphagia. Anastomotic leak rate between the esophagus and the conduit used for esophageal replacement is the highest among any surgical anastomosis, and is a dreaded complication because of its consequence. It remains a principle cause of surgical sepsis and its associated morbidity and mortality is high. The incidence of this complication varies widely but, even in the modern era in specialized centers, rates of around 10 % are still seen [1]. Stricture of the anastomosis, although generally easy to treat by endoscopic dilatation, generates anxiety for the cancer patient when it occurs, and has cost implications. Anastomotic recurrence is a difficult problem, since reoperation with tumor resection is often impossible after an esophagectomy.

These three problems associated with the esophageal anastomosis are largely technique-dependent. How one surgeon chooses a particular method depends as much on his/her preference and prior experience as on pure scientific evidence. It is the purpose of this article to review some of the many controversies with regard to esophageal anastomosis.

S. Law
Department of Surgery, Division of Esophageal and Upper Gastrointestinal Surgery,
The University of Hong Kong, Queen Mary Hospital,
102 Pokfulam Road,
Hong Kong, China
e-mail: slaw@hku.hk

12.2 Selection of Location of Anastomosis

Many considerations determine where the esophageal anastomosis is constructed. The location of the primary tumor is important. A cancer of the gastroesophageal junction with limited extension into the esophagus could have the anastomosis constructed in the lower mediastinum via an abdominal approach, or in the chest via a transthoracic method, or even in the neck. But a cancer of the superior mediastinal segment of the esophagus would dictate an anastomosis in the neck. An inadequate resection margin may result in a histologically involved margin, and hence subsequent recurrence. The propensity of esophageal cancer to spread intramurally and to have multiple disparate tumors is well recognized and contributes in part to such recurrence. The prevalence of intraepithelial or subepithelial spread was as high as 46 and 54 % in one report [2]. Our own pathologic study by serial sectioning of resected specimens showed a 26 % incidence of intramural metastasis [3]. The pattern of spread may vary with the depth of invasion of the primary lesion. Contiguous intraepithelial spread

L. Bonavina (ed.), *Innovation in Esophageal Surgery*,
DOI 10.1007/978-88-470-2469-4_12, © Springer-Verlag Italia 2012

frequently exists in early-stage cancer whereas subepithelial lesions are found in advanced cancer. The deeper the wall penetration of the primary tumor, the further away such spread can take place [2]. Some surgeons advocate routine subtotal esophagectomy with cervical anastomosis to attain the longest resection margin regardless of the site of the primary cancer. We have shown previously that the chance of anastomotic recurrence is a function of the length of proximal resection margin obtained at operation. In our patients, all patients who developed recurrences had a proximal margin of less than 5 cm [4]. Taking into account shrinkage of the specimen after resection [5], as a guide to surgery, an *in-situ* margin of approximately 10 cm should be the aim [4, 6].

In addition to the consideration of adequacy of the resection margin, the choice of surgical approach is another factor. Proponents of transhiatal resection would routinely perform cervical anastomosis [1]. Similarly if three-field lymphadenectomy is performed, then cervical anastomosis is a logical choice. If thoracoscopic or laparoscopic esophagectomy is carried out, then it is easier to perform cervical anastomosis rather than an intrathoracic one by minimally invasive methods. When a transthoracic open resection is performed, then either an intrathoracic anastomosis (Lewis Tanner esophagectomy), or a cervical esophagectomy (three-phase esophagectomy) can be done. In general, when an intrathoracic anastomosis is performed, the higher the level of anastomosis, the more desirable it is because of the increased resection margin, and also less gastroesophageal reflux symptoms result. In this regard, a narrower gastric tube makes "gastric retention" – and thus reflux – less likely.

The organ used for esophageal substitution influences the location of the anastomosis. When a gastroesophageal junction tumor involving the gastric cardia is resected with a substantial portion of the proximal stomach, the *distal* stomach when used as the conduit may not be able to reach the neck, thus dictating an intrathoracic esophagogastrostomy. When a colonic interposition is carried out, the anastomosis is usually in the neck to allow a straighter path. When a jejunal conduit is used, an intrathoracic (via a thoracotomy) or low mediastinal (using a stapler via a widened abdominal diaphragmatic hiatus) anastomosis is preferred because of the tedious and often difficult preparation of the loop to reach the neck, risking ischemia.

The surgeon's own anastomotic leak rate is also a determinant of the choice of anastomotic location because it is generally perceived that a cervical leak is easier to manage, and is less lethal compared to a thoracic leak; thus if a surgeon is plagued by a high leakage rate, a cervical anastomosis seems more appropriate. Unfortunately, the site of the esophageal anastomosis is also implicated as an important factor predisposing to leakage. Cervical anastomoses seem to have a higher tendency to leak compared to intrathoracic anastomoses. Less than 10 % of thoracic anastomoses, and 10–25 % of cervical anastomoses develop insufficiency [7]. A higher leakage rate in the neck may be due to a longer route used and hence tension created, and compression of the conduit at the thoracic inlet. In this respect the retrosternal route has higher leakage rates compared to the orthotopic route [8]. A recent meta-analysis comparing cervical or thoracic anastomosis after esophagectomy demonstrated a higher leak rate with cervical vs. thoracic anastomosis (19 vs. 5 %); there was a higher incidence of recurrent laryngeal nerve injury (17 vs. 3 %), but stricture rates were similar (14 vs. 15 %). The studies included however featured many cases in which cervical hand-sewn method was compared with an intrathoracic stapled anastomosis, so not only the location of the anastomosis varied, but also the method of construction [9].

This higher leak rate in the neck, however, is not universal. Similar leakage rates at the two sites have been reported by us and others [4, 10, 11]. In addition, a cervical leak may not be truly confined to the neck since mediastinal contamination from above is common. However, multivariate analysis in our patients did show a higher anastomotic stricture rate with cervical anastomosis [4].

12.3 Etiology of Leaks and Strictures: Technique of Esophageal Anastomosis

There are many theoretical reasons why the esophageal anastomosis is so prone to failure [7]. The esophagus is believed to be unfavorable anatomically for suturing; it has no serosa like the rest of the gastrointestinal tract, its longitudinal muscle holds sutures poorly, and the anastomosis is carried out in poorly exposed, awkward positions. Other local factors include vascular (both arterial and venous) insufficiency to the gastric fundus (the most commonly used esophageal substitute), tension at the anastomosis, gastric distension in the early postoperative period, and compression at the thoracic inlet compromising a cervical anastomosis. Systemic factors include severe malnutrition, hypoalbuminemia, and peri-operative hypoxia or hypotension.

That the esophageal wall is weak and does not hold sutures probably is not the main factor accounting for most anastomotic leaks. In the absence of tension at the anastomosis, its apparent *weakness* is not significant. The stomach is usually of ample length to reach the neck.

One important factor that contributes to leak is tissue ischemia; this is more likely from the conduit than the esophagus. The esophagus has a rich submucosal vascular network; this is evident from brisk bleeding often encountered at the esophageal edge when it is cut. The stomach usually has an adequate blood supply if it is prepared with care. A corrosion cast study of the gastric conduit showed that the stomach blood flow can rely on the right gastroepiploic artery alone, with the best blood supply to a 4 cm gastric tube on the greater curvature [12]. The right gastric artery can be divided if preservation results in tension to the esophago-gastric anastomosis. The colon's blood supply is more variable, but a pre-operative arteriogram may help in identifying reliable vasculature and lessen the risk of graft failure. Arterial anatomic features are favorable in at least 80 % of patients with arteriogram examination, and anastomotic leak rate and graft failure can be less than 2 % [13, 14].

Vascular insufficiency of the conduit may result if its preparation results in bruising or kinking of the supplying vessels resulting in ischemia. Clinically inapparent ischemia of the gastric fundus probably contributes to anastomotic failure. Various innovative methods have been proposed to improve vascular supply to the stomach tube. One method involves *ischemic pre-conditioning* of the gastric fundus to improve oxygenation. This is achieved by laparoscopic mobilization of the stomach followed by a staged-transthoracic resection [15, 16]. Unfortunately although working well in the laboratory and when mucosal oxygenation is measured [17], the technique remains disappointing in the clinical setting with similar leak rates compared to patients with no pre-conditioning [16]. Its value in routine use also seems limited since a low leak rate can be achieved using conventional anastomotic techniques anyway. The challenge may be to identify the appropriate patients for its selective application.

The esophageal anastomosis can be constructed with either a hand-sewn technique or by using the stapler, which can be a circular or a linear stapler. For hand anastomosis, a variety of methods are favored. The use of absorbable or non-absorbable, one- or two-layered, and continuous or interrupted sutures remains controversial [4, 8]. The results of most of these techniques are comparable.

Perceived advantages of using the stapled method are many, which include its ease of application when surgical exposure is suboptimal, such as at the apex of the chest or in the lower mediastinum when one approaches via the diaphragmatic hiatus from the abdomen. It is technically less operator-dependent, and the leak rate may be lower. Certainly, performing the anastomosis via the diaphragmatic hiatus in an obese patient with poor exposure is eased by use

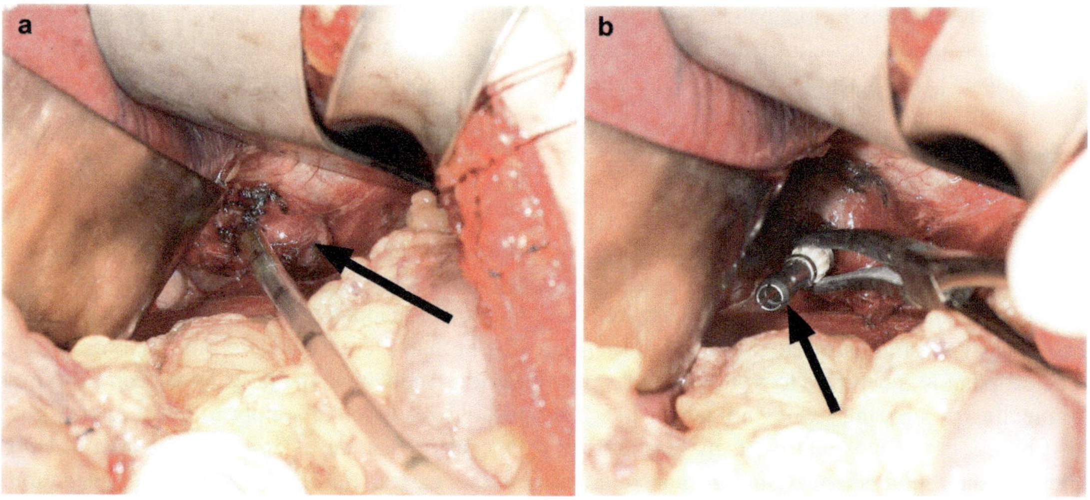

Fig. 12.1 Transoral placement of the anvil using the ORVIL device to ease application of the circular stapler (**a**) the ORVIL device emerging through a stapled esophageal stump in the lower medisatinum, arrow pointing at the esophageal stump (**b**) the anvil has been placed ready for anastomosis (*arrow*)

of a circular stapler; transoral placement of the anvil using the Orvil (Covidien) is of additional help (Fig. 12.1). In the author's experience, exposure at the apex of the chest is generally adequate for a hand-sewn anastomosis, with the exception that when poor one-lung anesthesia results (as frequently) in an obstructed view of the anastomosis, a stapled method can ease its construction. The circular stapler is awkward to use in the neck because of confined space. Many surgeons prefer to staple high thoracic anastomosis and suture cervical anastomosis.

An earlier pooled data analysis from randomized trials comparing stapled with hand-sewn esophagogastric anastomoses showed no significant difference for leaks (stapled 9 %, hand-sewn 8 %), but a higher incidence of strictures in stapled anastomoses (stapled 27 %, hand-sewn 16 %) [18]. A more recent systemic review addressing this issue showed that in eight randomized trials, out of 356 patients who underwent a hand-sewn anastomosis the leak rate was 8.9 % while it was 9.3 % in 354 patients who had a stapled anastomosis. The stricture rates did not show a significant difference at 15 and 26 % respectively [19]. Only one study conducted at the author's institution showed a significant difference in stricture rates, which were 9 vs. 40 % in hand-sewn and stapled groups respectively; the stapled cartridge size was also an important factor, with larger cartridge size resulting in less stenosis [20] (Fig. 12.2). One problem about the studies of stricture is that definitions of stricture were highly variable.

The linear stapler has also been used with success in some centers for anastomosis. One group reduced their clinically diagnosed cervical anastomotic leak rate from 14 % using a hand-sewn technique to 2.7 % using linear staples with a side-to-side anastomosis [1]. The stricture rate reduced from 48 to 35 %. In a recent single-center study involving 283 patients comparing three groups of patients with a hand-sewn method, circular stapler and a linear stapler, leak rates were no different at 3.4, 1.5 and 1.2 % respectively; however the diameters of the anastomosis measured by barium contrast study were 1.2, 1.5 and 1.6 cm, and stricture rates (defined as less than 0.8 cm on barium study) were 9.3, 20.9 and 1.9 %. Multivariate analysis identified age and anastomotic techniques as predictors of stricture development. Dysphagia score and reflux scores were all better in the linear stapler group [21]. The study was not randomized and biases existed in the selection of patients and the way stricture was defined, but the results were highly suggestive of less stricture formation using this linear stapled method.

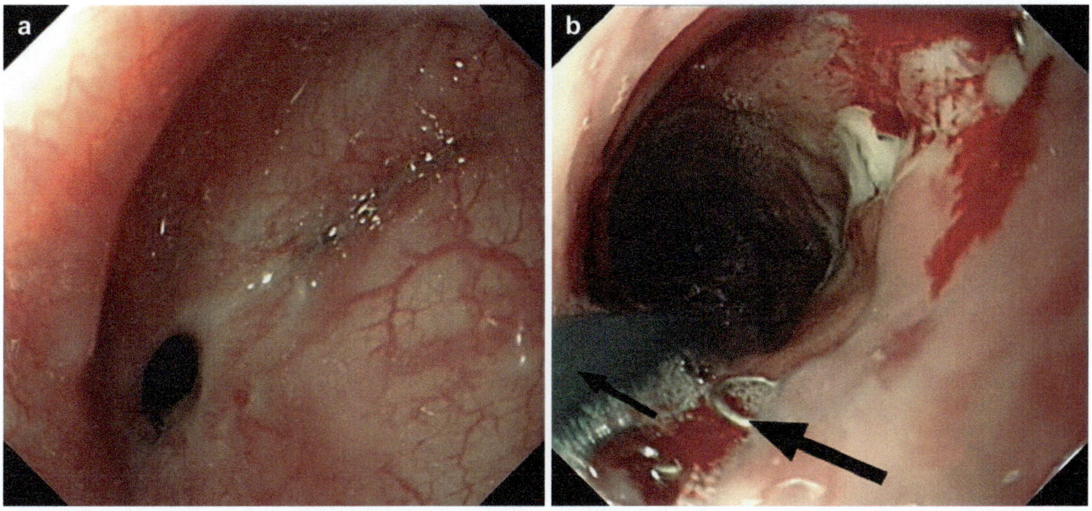

Fig. 12.2 (**a**) Endoscopic picture showing an anastomotic stricture 2 weeks after a circular stapled anastomosis. (**b**) This was treated by endoscopic dilatation. *Small arrow* pointing at the balloon dilator, *large arrow* pointing at the metallic staples

Another interesting finding showed that postoperative acid suppression could potentially lessen the chance of stricture formation, presumably by reducing esophagitis/inflammation at the anastomosis. A clinical trial was conducted in 80 patients who underwent circular stapled anastomosis, randomized to two groups with or without proton pump inhibitors (PPI). Those who had had prior chemotherapy, radiotherapy, and leaks after surgery were excluded. A stricture was defined as inability to pass a 9.2–9.5 mm endoscope with or without the symptom of dysphagia. The stricture rate was 43 % in those without medication and 13 % in those prescribed PPI. Cox regression showed that use of PPI and stapler cartridge size were independent predictors of outcome [22].

To further augment the anastomosis and reduce leak rates, other methods have been designed. These include covering the anastomoses with omentum, pleura, or pericardial fat, and using fibrin glue to spray the anastomosis. None have appeared reliable. Interestingly, two recent, very similar randomized trials were reported comparing patients with and without an omental pedicle flap around the esophago-gastric anastomosis. In the first study, 255 patients were randomized; all patients had a stapled anastomosis, and were stratified for a transthoracic or transhiatal esophagectomy. Leak rates were 0.8 vs. 5.5 % in those with or without omental wrap respectively ($p=0.03$); stricture rates were also significantly lower in the former group (6 vs. 16 %) [23]. In the second study, 194 patients were randomized, and also stratified for transhiatal or transthoracic resections. All patients had a manual anastomosis; leak rates were 3 % in the omental wrap group compared to 14 % in the group with no wrap; stricture rates however were no different at 10 and 7 % respectively [24]. The difference in hand-sewn and stapled anastomosis could be the reason why the influence on stricture rates was variable between the two studies.

Avoiding excessive blood loss during surgery, good pulmonary and cardiovascular support postoperatively to avoid hypoxia and hypotension are also important. Other inconstant factors predisposing to leakage include radiotherapy, chemotherapy, diabetes, age of patient, cirrhosis, and cardiopulmonary diseases [7]. Malignant infiltration of the esophageal resection margin was implicated in some studies [7, 25], but not in our own study; a positive resection margin was not found to predispose to anastomotic leak [6].

Technical errors probably account for most cases of anastomotic leaks. An analysis of our patients who underwent transthoracic resection over a 16-year period showed that of 17 leaks, at least one technical or surgical factor was identifiable that had the potential to contribute to leakage. For example, patients in the leak group were significantly more likely to have documented anastomotic technical difficulty, damage to the tracheobronchial tree, post-operative gastric outlet obstruction, or re-exploration for mediastinal hemorrhage [26]. A simple assessment of the surgeon at the end of surgery was a strong predictor of subsequent anastomotic leak: 53 % of leaks had an identifiable adverse factor intraoperatively [4].

The method of anastomosis is perhaps less important than its proper application. This applies whether the method of anastomosis is hand-sewn or stapled. In general, in experienced hands, the stapled and hand-sewn techniques give equivalent leakage rates. The stapled method may be less operator-dependent. With experience, results should improve. In the author's unit, leak rates used to be nearly 25 % between 1964 and 1982; thereafter they improved to less than 5 % and the rate is at present 3 % [4, 26, 27].

12.4 Anastomotic Leak: Diagnosis and Management

The principles of managing anastomotic leaks are: (1) early diagnosis; (2) adequate drainage; (3) antibiotics and control of sepsis; (4) nutritional support; and (5) sealing the leak if possible. Early fulminant leaks within the first 48 h are usually due to punctate necrosis or gangrene of the conduit. The patient may present with septicemia, and a large volume of foul chest tube discharge may be evident. Operative intervention is mandatory. The conduit should be taken down, appropriate debridement and drainage of the thoracic cavity and mediastinum established, a cervical esophagostomy performed and a feeding enterostomy done for nutritional support. Maximum esophageal length should be preserved to ease future reconstruction.

Clinically apparent thoracic leaks usually take place within the first week. A leak should be suspected in any patient who is not recovering adequately, e.g. in those who develop fever, tachycardia, arrhythmia, or poor arterial oxygenation. In our experience, onset of atrial arrhythmia may be an early indication of surgical sepsis, and a proactive search for a source, including anastomotic leak, is mandatory [28]. This may be confirmed by excessive output from the chest tube, which may be turbid in color or bile-stained. Pleural collections on chest radiograph or computed tomography (CT) scans may be evident. Confirmation can be obtained by giving the patient methylene blue dye orally and observing this dye as it appears in the chest drainage. The location and magnitude of the leak can be visualized by a water-soluble contrast study. A carefully performed flexible endoscopic examination is also helpful to appreciate the site and size of leakage and should not aggravate the leak if done carefully. The treatment of anastomotic leaks should be individualized. For small contained leaks, conservative observation may suffice. In septic patients with a sizable leak, exploration is warranted. Direct repair is rarely successful. In selected patients, a combination of endoscopically guided nasogastric tube placement for decompression, naso-cavity drain for collection drainage, and naso-jejunal tube for nutritional support, with or without radiologically guided percutaneous drainage, can be successful without the need for surgical re-exploration. Other minimally invasive techniques have been described, such as combining endoscopic and thoracoscopic placement of T-tube for drainage [29], or endoscopic placement of transnasal draining tubes, armed with a size-adjusted sponge at their distal end, in the necrotic anastomotic cavities, followed by continuous suction. This latter method however does require multiple procedures and only applies to large leaks [30].

For a cervical anastomosis, leakage is suspected when there is inflammation and pain of the neck wound. Turbid infected discharge is found when the skin stitches are removed. Leaks truly confined to the neck are simply treated by laying the wound open with daily washing and frequent change of dressing. The patient is usually not septic. Leaks that communicate with the mediastinum may require formal exploration and placement of mediastinal drains.

A more recently employed technique is the use of covered stents to occlude the fistula. These can be metallic [31] or plastic stents [32]. Success in fistula occlusion is generally high (>90 %), with control of sepsis, earlier alimentation, and shorter intensive care and hospital stay [32], although misplacement of stent may worsen the clinical situation, such as enlarging the leak. A recent series using plastic stents in 22 patients achieved success in 21; however, in 13 of these repeated stenting was necessary, and migrations occurred in 5 [33]. Migration rate can be up to 40 %. Stent harvesting from the patients' excrement has been reported [31]. Certainly stent insertion for leak occlusion is an attractive minimally invasive option. It is more suitable for intrathoracic than cervical leaks; the short proximal esophagus in the latter situation does not provide enough room for stent purchase and in theory migration is more likely.

Subclinical leaks detected by contrast study only may be treated conservatively. Follow up contrast study is done to monitor healing. Treatment is modified if clinical sepsis occurs or radiologic progression takes place. Drainage should also be considered in leaks close to the trachea or aorta, as broncho-gastric fistulation has been reported [34].

Treatment of anastomotic leaks has improved over the years. At the author's institute, leakage rate from 1964 to 1982 was 16, and 61 % of these patients died, making an overall leak-related mortality rate of 9.8 % [27]. From 1982 to 1998, the leakage rate was 3.5, and 35 % of patients died, giving a leak-related mortality rate of 1.2 % [26]. In recent years (1996–2002), the corresponding figures were 3.2, 0 and 0 %. Surgical experience should lead to lower leakage rates. A high index of suspicion, and timely diagnosis and intervention will lower mortality rate from this feared complication of esophageal surgery.

Key Points

- Location of tumor and method of resection dictate the choice of anastomotic site
- Stapled and hand-sewn anastomotic techniques are equally safe
- Leak to a large extent is technique-dependent
- Stricture is esophageal size- and technique-dependent
- Aggressive and early proactive treatment of leaks ensures good outcome
- Mortality from leak should be uncommon

References

1. Orringer MB, Marshall B, Chang AC et al (2007) Two thousand transhiatal esophagectomies: changing trends, lessons learned. Ann Surg 246(3):363–372
2. Tsutsui S, Kuwano H, Watanabe M et al (1995) Resection margin for squamous cell carcinoma of the esophagus. Ann Surg 222(2):193–202
3. Lam KY, Ma LT, Wong J (1996) Measurement of extent of spread of oesophageal squamous carcinoma by serial sectioning. J Clin Pathol 49:124–129
4. Law S, Suen DT, Wong KH et al (2005) A single-layer, continuous, hand-sewn method for esophageal anastomosis: prospective evaluation in 218 patients. Arch Surg 140(1):33–39
5. Siu KF, Cheung HC, Wong J (1986) Shrinkage of the esophagus after resection for carcinoma. Ann Surg 203(2):173–176
6. Law S, Arcilla C, Chu KM et al (1998) The significance of histologically infiltrated resection margin after esophagectomy for esophageal cancer. Am J Surg 176:286–290
7. Urschel JD (1995) Esophagogastrostomy anastomotic leaks complicating esophagectomy: a review. Am J Surg 169:634–640
8. Zieren HU, Muller JM, Pichlmaier H (1993) Prospective randomized study of one- or two-layer anastomosis following oesophageal resection and cervical oesophagogastrostomy. Br J Surg 80(5):608–611
9. Biere SS, Maas KW, Cuesta MA et al (2011) Cervical or thoracic anastomosis after esophagectomy for cancer: a systematic review and meta-analysis. Dig Surg 28(1):29–35
10. Goldfaden D, Orringer MB, Appelman HD et al (1986) Adenocarcinoma of the distal esophagus and gastric cardia: comparison of results of transhiatal esophagectomy and thoracoabdominal esophagogastrectomy. J Thorac Cardiovasc Surg 91:242–247

11. Lam TC, Fok M, Cheng SW et al (1992) Anastomotic complications after esophagectomy for cancer. A comparison of neck and chest anastomoses. J Thorac Cardiovasc Surg 104(2):395–400
12. Liebermann-Meffert DMI, Meier R, Siewert JR (1992) Vascular anatomy of the gastric tube used for esophageal reconstruction. Ann Thorac Surg 54: 1110–1115
13. Peters JH, Kronson JW, Katz M et al (1995) Arterial anatomic considerations in colon interposition for esophageal replacement. Arch Surg 130:858–863
14. Davis PA, Law S, Wong J (2003) Colonic interposition after esophagectomy for cancer. Arch Surg 138(3):303–308
15. Holscher AH, Schneider PM, Gutschow C et al (2007) Laparoscopic ischemic conditioning of the stomach for esophageal replacement. Ann Surg 245(2):241–246
16. Schroder W, Holscher AH, Bludau M et al (2010) Ivor-Lewis esophagectomy with and without laparoscopic conditioning of the gastric conduit. World J Surg 34(4):738–743
17. Bludau M, Holscher AH, Vallbohmer D et al (2010) Ischemic conditioning of the gastric conduit prior to esophagectomy improves mucosal oxygen saturation. Ann Thorac Surg 90(4):1121–1126
18. Urschel JD, Blewett CJ, Bennett WF et al (2001) Handsewn or stapled esophagogastric anastomoses after esophagectomy for cancer: meta-analysis of randomized controlled trials. Dis Esophagus 14(3–4):212–217
19. Kim RH, Takabe K (2010) Methods of esophagogastric anastomoses following esophagectomy for cancer: a systematic review. J Surg Oncol 101(6): 527–533
20. Law S, Fok M, Chu KM et al (1997) Comparison of hand-sewn and stapled esophagogastric anastomosis after esophageal resection for cancer: a prospective randomized controlled trial. Ann Surg 226(2):169–173
21. Xu QR, Wang KN, Wang WP et al (2011) Linear stapled esophagogastrostomy is more effective than hand-sewn or circular stapler in prevention of anastomotic stricture: a comparative clinical study. J Gastrointest Surg 15(6):915–921
22. Johansson J, Oberg S, Wenner J et al (2009) Impact of proton pump inhibitors on benign anastomotic stricture formations after esophagectomy and gastric tube reconstruction: results from a randomized clinical trial. Ann Surg 250(5):667–673
23. Dai JG, Zhang ZY, Min JX et al (2011) Wrapping of the omental pedicle flap around esophagogastric anastomosis after esophagectomy for esophageal cancer. Surgery 149(3):404–410
24. Bhat MA, Dar MA, Lone GN et al (2006) Use of pedicled omentum in esophagogastric anastomosis for prevention of anastomotic leak. Ann Thorac Surg 82(5):1857–1862
25. Patil PK, Patel SG, Mistry RC et al (1992) Cancer of the esophagus: esophagogastric anastomotic leak- a retrospective study of predisposing factors. J Surg Oncol 49(3):163–167
26. Whooley BP, Law S, Alexandrou A et al (2001) Critical appraisal of the significance of intrathoracic anastomotic leakage after esophagectomy for cancer. Am J Surg 181(3):198–203
27. Lorentz T, Fok M, Wong J (1989) Anastomotic leakage after resection and bypass for esophageal cancer: lessons learned from the past. World J Surg 13(4):472–477
28. Murthy SC, Law S, Whooley BP et al (2003) Atrial fibrillation after esophagectomy is a marker for postoperative morbidity and mortality. J Thorac Cardiovasc Surg 126(4):1162–1167
29. Nguyen NT, Hinojosa MW, Fayad C et al (2007) Minimally invasive management of intrathoracic leaks after esophagogastrectomy. Surg Innov 14(2):96–101
30. Wedemeyer J, Brangewitz M, Kubicka S et al (2010) Management of major postsurgical gastroesophageal intrathoracic leaks with an endoscopic vacuum-assisted closure system. Gastrointest Endosc 71(2): 382–386
31. Kauer WKH, Stein HJ, Dittler HJ, Siewert JR Stent implantation as a treatment option in patients with thoracic anastomotic leaks after esophagectomy Surg Endosc 2008;22:50–53
32. Hunerbein M, Stroszczynski C, Moesta KT et al (2004) Treatment of thoracic anastomotic leaks after esophagectomy with self-expanding plastic stents. Ann Surg 240(5):801–807
33. Dai YY, Gretschel S, Dudeck O et al (2009) Treatment of oesophageal anastomotic leaks by temporary stenting with self-expanding plastic stents. Br J Surg 96(8):887–891
34. Mok VW, Ting AC, Law S et al (2004) Combined endovascular stent grafting and endoscopic injection of fibrin sealant for aortoenteric fistula complicating esophagectomy. J Vasc Surg 40(6):1234–1237

Rationale and Outcomes of the Kaizen Method Applied to Esophagectomy

13

Mark D. Iannettoni

13.1 Introduction

Medicine has always been taught historically as an art form rather than an exact science with a unpredictable outcome due to the infinite variability associated with human physiology. However, with the advancements in medicine and the use of evidence-based medicine as well as outcome studies, we are more able to predict and model our current practices and methods. Most surgical experience and current methods involve the past practice of our teachers and are based on what we know works rather than what we can prove.

If one looks at complex industrial processes we see there are several opportunities to apply these principles to a wide array of surgical interventions and processes in an attempt to improve outcomes, reduce variability and, as a by-product, reduce costs. The most expensive part of any surgical intervention is the cost of a complication, which results in additional intervention for the patients, cost for the hospital, an increase in length of stay (LOS) and delayed return to the workforce or meaningful lifestyle [1]. By limiting variability and following principles applied to operations engineering and, most importantly, having the willingness to change the way things are done based on certain applied criteria, we are able to control this variability and improve outcomes while reducing costs.

The idea of *fast tracking* in thoracic surgery is not a new concept for us since our first attempt to describe this endeavor was with outpatient thoracoscopy in 2002. Unfortunately, our initial description of fast tracking did not relay the appropriate message that we wanted to deliver by these concepts [2].

Our later attempts to refine this description really relate to process analysis, operations engineering and continuous improvement methods which result in improved outcomes, less variability and, as a by-product of these efforts, reduced costs as well as improved patient satisfaction. To this end we have used Kaizen methodology to improve the overall process of an esophagectomy from the initial patient visit to the final outpatient visit.

Kaizen methodology has been well documented in the literature and has been described eloquently by many others [3], but in brief the Japanese term *kaizen* literally means "improvement". This word, however, has been turned into a process by Western cultures and developed into a philosophy of continuous improvements by attempting to apply scientific methods to a series of complex processes. This analysis can be applied to almost any process, system, or event that can be operationalized. We attempted to apply this to a complex operative intervention, as well as analyzing our pre-operative and post-operative courses

M.D. Iannettoni
Department of Cardiothoracic Surgery,
University of Iowa Hospitals and Clinics,
200 Hawkins Drive SE514 GH, Iowa City,
IA 52242, USA
e-mail: mark-iannettoni@uiowa.edu

L. Bonavina (ed.), *Innovation in Esophageal Surgery*,
DOI 10.1007/978-88-470-2469-4_13, © Springer-Verlag Italia 2012

and events to hopefully improve outcomes, overall results and the patient experience. It is important to stress that the goal was not to reduce costs.

While other methods of operational improvements, such as Six Sigma, Lean or Just-in-Time methodology, were evaluated, these all had a flaw that once a system was identified, the changes were made and set from either a management perspective, cost perspective, or a way to reduce defects perspective, that can be control. These, however, are not continuous improvement projects and are not very conducive to being altered on the fly. They also remove the human element as a variable; not something we really desire in our patient care. More importantly none of these other methods really care about patient satisfaction, which was one of the goals of our project. These other methods may be good for inventory but not very good for patients.

In attempting to develop a Kaizen event one must identify the goals of the project up front to help guide the analysis, but also be willing to make changes to along the way to adjust for new findings or unrecognized opportunities for improvement. While stated earlier, it bears repeating multiple times that the Kaizen event is an event which allows and requires constant change to achieve the desired effect of continuous process improvement.

The utilization of the kaizen tool as it relates to esophagectomy was born out of necessity to provide process improvement, standardization of a complex procedure and the need for improved patient satisfaction for a difficult process. It is relatively unusual in any other field except surgery that a complex process or system is developed, determined and led by only one person who has the sole authority to dictate and direct these processes, that being the surgeon. Only rarely is this authority questioned, let alone challenged, by anyone in or out of the operating room. However, in other complex systems such as aviation, engineering processes, or even on the assembly line, the concept or understanding that being questioned or halting the process when something seems wrong or a possible problem is identified is not only the expectation but the obligation of everyone on the team. Surgery, on the other hand, has never been in step with this concept and for good reason. But, as in many cases where the immediacy of the situation requires these types of unfaltering response, similar to the military, after the fact, reconstructing the events with a breakdown of the events and subsequent analysis is never done.

The goals of our Kaizen event were to:

- improve patient outcomes;
- improve patient satisfaction;
- improve efficiency;
- standardize the process;
- limit variability;
- avoid waste.

In order to evaluate the process we as a group of health care providers looked at our total process of esophagectomy and broke it down into phases of care for each component to affect change at multiple levels of care [4]. These identified phases of care were as follows:

- initial contact;
- preoperative phase;
- intraoperative phase;
- postoperative phase;
- outpatient phase.

13.2 Initial Contact Phase

During the initial contact phase in the pre-Kaizen era we had an open access procedure with very little physician involvement or evaluation of the quality, quantity or standardization of the type of information required for entry of a patient into the system. An intake sheet was developed during our Kaizen discussions with our nursing staff to allow development of a standard tool to be used for entry into the clinic to reduce the number of visits a patient would have to make, which went from 4 to 7 visits on average depending on whether or not these visits needed to be coordinated with other care providers to only one surgical visit for all of the testing and pre-operative assessment (Fig. 13.1). This pre-operative checklist also allowed for standardized testing to be scheduled, resulting in a more uniform and cost conscious evaluation. The initial contact review also allowed for consultations to be scheduled prior to the visit or during the same visit if needed, reducing the number of visits back to our institution. This is an

Thoracic Surgery/ New Esophageal Date: ________ Appt: Date: ____________________ Referring MD______________________________ ______________________________	Name: Hospital #: Age:
CC:	SH: Tobacco use: Alcohol use: Occupation:
PMH:	FH:
Medications:	Allergies: Steroid use: Anticoagulation (ASA, Coumadin Plavix) STOP DATE:______________________
Plan/Procedure :	

Ordered/Reviewed		*Test*	*Date*	*Ordered/Reviewed*		*Test*	*Date*
☐	☐	Chest/ Abdominal CT				Pre-op	
☐	☐	Barium Swallow		☐	☐	CXR	
☐	☐	EGD with bx		☐	☐	EKG	
☐	☐	pH Testing		☐	☐	Labs	
☐	☐	Manometry		☐	☐	Consent/orders done	
☐	☐	EUS		☐	☐	Bed ordered	
☐	☐	PET		☐	☐	PICC done	
☐	☐	Barium Enema					
☐	☐	Outside path slides here					
☐	☐	PFT's					

MLH 2003

Fig. 13.1 New patient intake sheet

important consideration since many of our patients travel great distances to visit for consultation and planning.

This initial contact also gave us the opportunity to set expectations for the patients, their families and the referring physicians as to how this process was to play out. Providing this framework for patients reduced the anxiety of the visit and set the expectation that they may or may not be at the institution for the entire day; as well it allowed them some control of the process by helping to arrange for separate visits if desired or providing a one-stop experience.

13.3 Pre-operative Phase

Prior to the Kaizen event there was very little information review and this was done during the initial clinic visit which resulted in significant delays in complex patients due to duplicate testing if the information was not available, even if it had been gathered elsewhere. Attempting to ferret out the information on the day of the visit resulted in significant dissatisfaction, not only for the provider who may not have the information needed, but also for patients who might have had the testing done but had either not been asked to bring it with them or had to repeat the test. Having all of this material at hand and previously reviewed resulted in significantly more efficient and functional clinics, as well as providing the patient with a sense of satisfaction at being seen on time by a physician who already knew their information and understood their disease process and needs. More importantly, a clear plan could be established rather than the need for further testing or duplicate testing.

At this pre-operative phase, if needed we established appointments with oncology and radiation therapy to complete the patient's evaluation, and, if not, pre-operative testing was done and the patient was given an operative date. At this time patient education was also performed and information about their upcoming surgery, testing, anesthesia evaluation, and consenting was also performed so that the only thing to do prior to surgery was an update the morning of surgery and no further visits were required.

13.4 Operative Phase

One of the most challenging phases of any surgical procedure to standardize is the operative phase. Much of this is due to deep rooted training paradigms, and the unwillingness to change what seems to be working regardless of the evidence-based observations to the contrary. However, the two most expensive parts of most surgical interventions involve the operating room and the management of complications associated with variability in the operative or post-operative phase.

In this section we focus on the operative phase and attempts to reduce variability through evidence-based observations from our institution. It is important to note that these are observations from our predetermined ideals and what has worked and continues to be modified for our institution. Simply applying these operative methods to another institution will be fraught with poor outcomes unless the procedures and methodology already exist at another intuition. It is important to understand the difference between uniform practice and standardized practice. Uniform practice requires that all procedures are done the same way by all concerned. This is not always possible and may or may not result in the best outcomes. Standardized practice results from constant evaluation of process improvement and may result in uniform practice, but is simply evaluating a practice pattern that results in the best outcomes at all times. In short, uniform practice tries to make everyone the same; standardization tries to obtain the best results. An example is that practice doesn't make perfect, perfect practice makes perfect.

Prior to our Kaizen evaluation we had three different surgeons performing three different techniques with significant variability of results. During our intra-operative phase evaluation we looked at multiple variables from the operating room such as case duration, charges and costs, anesthetic requirements and resource utilization. We then compared these with outcomes and LOS data, as well as overall results and patient satisfaction.

By refining this process we were then able to standardize our operative technique and reduce operative variability from a historic 348 min to an average of 189 min (Table 13.1). This resulted from standardizing not only our technique but also scripting the events of the operation for all to see and follow. This resulted in significantly less variability, as well as limiting the cost of unused or unneeded supplies being added to the case carts. While supplies produce most of the cost, the most expensive part of the operating room is the time assigned for each procedure and the expense associated with the operation.

Operating room time can be calculated in a number of ways as to whether or not it is simply assigned to the room or whether this cost includes the anesthetic time as well. The range for this cost can be extremely variable but in general it ranges from approximately $45–$72/min. So while it is important to control the expense of staplers and additional devices, if the addition of newer technology, which costs $300 to open, can reduce operating time by 25 min, this results in a net savings of over $800 on the low end and $1,500 per case on the high end. These types of value decisions should be based on data-driven outcomes and surgical preference, not hospital economics. In other words, even though less expensive on a cost per case basis, if the result is more complications or increased LOS, the results must all be weighed up together.

Table 13.1 Comparison of operative phase

Pre Kaizen	Post Kaizen
Three different surgeons	Three different surgeons
Three different techniques	One technique
Three different intraoperative methods	Standardized anesthetic technique
Different anesthetic requests	Standardized operative equipment and disposables
Variable intraoperative supplies	Scripted intraoperative events
Average time: 348 min	Average time: 189 min

We have found that a well scripted surgical event is relatively easy to develop and it is readily adopted by the operating room staff and eventually by the physicians (Fig. 13.2). This is also an excellent training tool for our residents in developing organizational skills, as well as conduct of the operating room. It also limits the delay with new nursing trainees who may not be familiar with our system and allows them to be more procedurally directed rather than bound to on-the-job training, which has occurred in the past and increases time, cost and frustration to the operating surgeons.

13.5 Post-operative Phase

The changes in the post-operative phase really are the events that resulted in the change in our patient satisfaction issues. The major events that resulted in these improvements were not so much the events themselves but setting the stage and expectations well before the admission to hospital. Establishing the expectations for the patients and their families is the key role of the coordinator (to be discussed later); however, this is what makes the system work and how the patients know what to expect and react to their hospital stay.

The changes made in the post-operative phase have been the result of combined experience from different perspectives on what is needed and a combined management model for patients.

ABDOMINAL - PHASE I
GASTRIC MOBILIZATION
- bovie 50/50 (blend 1)
- upper hand retractor
- 2-0 long silk ties

PYLOROMYOTOMY
- bovie down to 40/40 (blend 1)
- dry laps x 2 folded in half
- 3-0 silk BB x 2
- 3-0 silk ties on mosquito available short rt. angle, diss. mosquito, coronary sxn
- ligaclips x 2 to mark site

J-TUBE (14fr robinson)
- 4-0 prolene RB-1 x 2 for pursestring & Weitzel

NECK – PHASE I
NECK INCISION (encircling esophagus)
- dry laps x 2
- adson x 2, short rt. angle x 2, army-navy x 1
- 3-0 short silk ties on mosquitoes
- 5-8" penrose/semb around cervical esophagus w/ medium snap

ESOPHAGEAL MOBILIZATION
- "finger" = metal yankauer tip
- sponge stick x 2 (1/2 raytec, moist)
- 28fr saratoga sump

TRANSECTING CERV. ESOPH.
- GIA 60/3.8
- allis clamp x 1 on remaining esoph.
- thoracic pk. w/ russian
- moist lap

Fig. 13.2 Example of scripted operative technique

Traditionally, care has been provided in a consistent manner with what has been done in the past. Changing these perspectives and perceptions on what must happen was difficult at first; however, as more data-driven care was provided, we found that these changes were not only safe but resulted in improved outcomes and patient satisfaction scores for our patient population.

Many of these decisions were a domino effect of changes made initially and then moving things forward with a constant process improvement method, which is the essence of a Kaizen event. The initial decision to extubate these patients in the operating room was aided by input from our anesthesia team who felt these patients really only had a significant insult with an upper midline incision and we would not routinely keep these patients intubated. The original concern was that these people could not protect their own airway well and many were insensate. The more important issue was that reintubation in these patients was usually catastrophic. In looking into why patients required reintubation after extubation, it was usually related to some complicating factor; however, this rarely occurred early on in the patient's hospital course; it was usually 2–3 days into the post-operative period. Therefore, a trial of extubation was done in the operating room and observation was performed to see if there were significant issues. There were, however, only a few cases that required reintubation and once our system was completely understood and our anesthesia colleagues were attuned to these patients, routine extubation has been the norm and no immediate reintubations have been encountered in any of those patients who were felt to be candidates for extubation.

The next step was to eliminate the Intensive Care Unit (ICU) stay for these patients. As they were not intubated, simple observation in the ICU was no longer needed. However, significant education of our regular nursing units was required as this was a significant change in practice. Nurses were educated by our coordinator as to what areas of concern would need to be identified and critical pathways were used to provide uniform care and reduce variability of the patient's course.

The reduction in hospital stay was a result of attempting to apply much of what we have learned with minimally invasive surgery, and then moving this model toward our transhiatal procedure. In the past we had routinely fed our patients at 3 days based on the assumption that they were swallowing 1–2 l of saliva a day regardless of their nasogastric tube. This worked reasonably well for most patients; however, as time has gone by we have seen a dramatic increase in our leak rate from 3 to 12 % based on several factors, mostly related to the increased use of chemotherapy and radiation. After a discussion with our otolaryngology colleagues in which we learned that many groups who routinely performed upper pharyngeal anastomoses did not feed patients for almost 4 weeks, we decided to adopt a non-randomized approach similar to this method and picked 15 days as our threshold to feeding. This was not completely an arbitrary number, but based on limited evidence in the literature. With this approach we have reduced our leak rate to one patient with an emergent operation for a perforated stricture on over 150 procedures, of which over 70 % have had pre-operative neoadjuvant therapy.

Strict adherence to care maps at our institution has resulted in a significant improvement in care, as well as a more well-scripted plan for patients and families, since everyone on the team - from residents to nurses to social worker and dietitian - understands how the system works and knows where the patient is in their course, so they can all provide their prospective care and planning for discharge which is routinely at 5 days (Fig. 13.3).

13.6 Nurse Coordinator

As much as we would like to think this is a physician-driven process, one of the key things the Kaizen event has brought to light is that while physician involvement in the process is key to the operative success of the procedure, it is the nurse coordinator who is in control of the overall perception that the patient will have. From the initial encounter either with the patient, the patient's

MULTIDISCIPLINARY CAREMAP

ESOPHAGECTOMY

Map ID No. 06105
Page 1

DATE
HOSP. NO.
NAME
BIRTH DATE
ADDRESS

IF NOT IMPRINTED, PLEASE PRINT DATE, HOSP. NO., NAME AND LOCATION

CRITICAL PATH (Care plan on reverse side)

	Pre-op Clinic Visit	POST OP: Day 0-2	POD 3-5
Interim Goals	Patient identifies acceptable pain level (pain scale 0-10) States name and purpose of medications	Pain at or below acceptable level $SaO_2 \geq 92\%$ Incision edges approximated without signs/symptoms of infection, drainage, erythema	Pain at or below acceptable level $SaO_2 \geq 92\%$ Incision edges approximated without signs/symptoms of infection, drainage, erythema Verbalizes understanding of discharge instructions States name/purpose of medications Demonstrates how to give medication via jejunostomy tube
Consults	Anesthesia visit Social Service PRN Smoking Cessation	Physical Therapy PRN Dietician Smoking Cessation PRN Respiratory Therapy PRN Pain Service PRN OT PRN Social Service PRN	VNA PRN Social Services PRN placement
Tests	History & Physical Consent signed EKG within 2 months unless chest pain or indicated CXR PA/LAT within 1 month Labs: CBC, PTT/pt/INR T&C in AM of OR	CGB q 6hr if diabetic CBC postop day 1 Schedule Barium Swallow for day #5	POD#5: Barium Swallow
Treatments/ Interventions	Vitals, ht & wt Skin Assessment Spirometry SCD only	VS q 4hr Bilat Chest tube @ 20 cm LCS and output q8 hr Epidural per Pain Service Foley to SD Penrose drain with dry dsg q 8 hr & PRN Jejunostomy tube: To gravity flush Jejunostomy tube w/20cc of NS q 4 hrs NG: to LCS flush w/30 cc tap H_2O q 8 hr I&O q 8 hr; call if UO<250cc q8 hr TCDB q1 while awake; IS q 1 hr while awake Oral Care: 4x per/day w/toothbrush, Yankour to sux secretions PRN Telemetry O_2 per nc, wean to keep sats >88% Pain assessment q 4 hr & PRN SCD while in BED Daily wts @ 0800	VS q 8 hr POD#3: DC chest tube or when output <150cc x2 shifts POD #3: DC Epidural POD #3-4: DC Penrose drain POD #3: Jejunostomy tube feedings per Dietician POD #4: DC NG I&O q 8 hr; call if UO <250 cc q8 hr TCDB q 1while awake; IS q 1 hr while awake Oral Care: 4xper/day w/toothbrush Telemetry: DC O_2 per nc, wean to keep sats >88% Pain assessment q 4 hr & PRN SCD while in BED Daily wts @ 0800 Remove neck sutures before discharge or Day #10
Medications	Medications taken preop per anesthesia instructions	IV fluids: per MD order Medications: per MD order Heparin 5000 units SQ q 12 hr	POD#3: Hold AM Heparin for Epidural DC Peridex 5 ml. Oral swab QID
Diet	NPO after Midnight	Ice chips : Max 30 cc/shift	POD #1NPO-Day #15 POD#3: Initiate Jejunostomy tube Feedings per Dietician Increase to Goal not to exceed 75cc/hr
Activity	UAL as tolerated	HOB up 45 degrees at all time Aspiration precautions Neck Flex at 45 degrees at all times Ambulate increased to QID Chair TID	HOB up 45 degrees at all time Aspiration precautions Neck Flex at 45 degrees at all times Ambulate increased to QID Chair TID
Teaching	Preop Teaching Post-op pain control Esophogeal surgery booklet		Post Esophagectomy Care Medications Return Appointment Jejunostomy tube feedings instructions PRN Mushy soft diet instructions
Discharge Planning	Asess home needs, teaching needs Home health nurse Social Service Transportation	Start VNA referral	Home going med prescriptions VNA referral and call VNA Scripts for equipment RTC appointment at 1 month Discharge with PT order x 3 weeks, if needed

Fig. 13.3 Care map for esophagectomy

family or the referring physician's office, the impression established by the nurse coordinator is key to the success of the future encounter (Fig. 13.4). How well we present ourselves prior to the patient's arrival is one of the most meaningful things we have discovered in how we establish the patient's expectations. It is then our job to meet or exceed these expectations with the

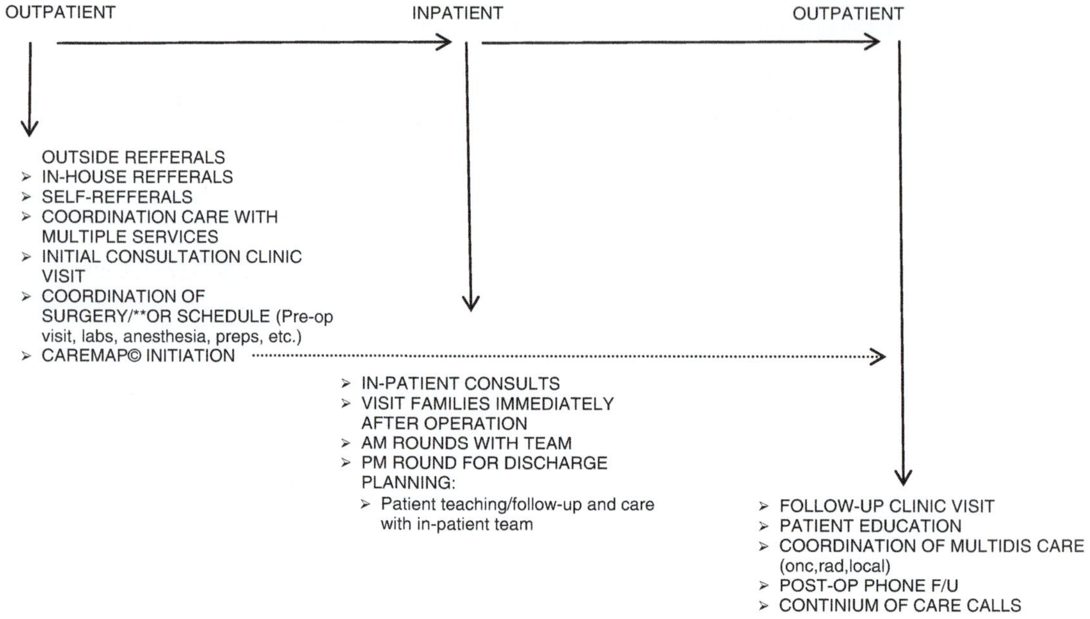

Fig. 13.4 The nurse coordinator role

service we provide, both as care providers and how we listen to our customers. The nurse coordinator has the dual role of providing for the needs of the patients, but also carrying out the plan set forth by the physicians and the care teams with respect to the operation being performed.

It is this important link provided by the nurse coordinator that puts patients at ease with the process at hand prior to their visit, as well as letting them know they have a consistent and constant resource after the procedure, that allows this early discharge planning and solid communication for patients and their families. While this is a significant workload and added expense for any program, the result in decreased LOS and preventing readmissions rapidly outweighs any increase in cost. More importantly, the patient experience is markedly improved, as demonstrated by the marked increase in our patient satisfaction scores.

13.7 Unintended Consequences

The Kaizen event has many unintended consequences and requires the ability of physicians, as well as the administration, to be willing to change their current practice paradigms and show a true willingness for change. Some of these unintended consequences are good and some are opportunities for improvement.

While the hope for a Kaizen event is improved care in our industry, it may come at the expense of profits initially, as it may require the addition of personnel, where identified, to improve throughput, standardization, patient care or discharge planning. Ultimately, however, this standardized approach should result in efficiencies that improve LOS, cost and patient satisfaction (Table 13.2).

We have demonstrated significant cost savings, mostly from a reduction in operating room time and standardization of post-operative care plans (Table 13.3). However, the cost of adding a nurse coordinator or two is not insignificant, so one must look at the volume, current cost and outcomes and be careful to track these changes to see the effect of Kaizen efforts to truly demonstrate improvements in health care delivery. The intangible of improved patient satisfaction by delivery of outstanding healthcare and the care provided by the nurse coordinator can be measured in not only improved outcomes but a volume increase due to referrals of new patients

Table 13.2 Overall changes associated with our Kaizen event

Pre Kaizen	Post Kaizen
ICU stay intubated	Extubated in the OR
LOS initially 14 days	No ICU stay
Invasive monitoring	No invasive monitoring
Due to operative variability	LOS 5 days
Leak rate 12 %	Strict adherence to care maps
Limited documentation for postoperative planning	No leaks in last 64 consecutive patients

Table 13.3 Overall cost reduction due to Kaizen methodology

Charges*	Pre-Kaizen	Post-Kaizen
ICU – accommodation charge	$3,810.00	$0.00
1 day ventilator	1,228.00	0.00
1 day general care w/monitor	15,435.00	6,615.00
1 day on the floor w/o monitor	9,940.00	2,840.00
Blood gases	546.00	0.00
CXR AP – one view	732.00	244.00
CXR AP – two view	1,395.00	279.00
CBC, chem. Profile and electrolytes – average	704.00	88.00
Cost of 1 min of OR time with anesthesia costs included:		
Category 5 – base	3,538.00	3,538.00
Category 5 – per min	21,454.20	11,651.85
Anesthesia materials – major base charge (multiple base charges can be incurred based on complexity of surgery)	816.00	408.00
Anesthesia materials – major (per min charge)	2,105.40	1,361.25
*Adjusted for 2009 dollars	$61,703.60	$27,025.10
Cost savings	**$34,678.50**	**43.80 %**

seeking the same experience and this attention to detail provided by the nurse coordinator. Needless to say, the right person in this role can make or break the experience, so treat them well!

13.8 Summary

The complex nature of surgical interventions and the intricacies of performing these complex tasks greatly lend themselves to intense analysis of the process by a team approach. This systematic team approach to these complex systems would result in the best outcomes for the patients as well as improved efficiencies, and most likely reduced costs [5]. However we continue on a path of individualization with respect to health care and patient management, which interjects variability into the process, which results in decreased efficiency for the team at best and unpredictable results at worst. While we all recognize that each patient is an individual and should be treated as such, the patient experience for a standardized procedure should be the same for all patients and should result in similar outcomes and improved overall care.

Key Points

- Principles derived from complex industrial processes can be applied to a wide array of surgical interventions in an attempt to improve outcomes, reduce variability, and reduce costs
- Cost of a complication is the most expensive part of surgical interventions for esophageal cancer
- A systematic team approach and practice standardization according to Kaizen methodology has the potential to improve the outcome of esophagectomy

References

1. Dimick JB, Chen SL, Taheri PA et al (2004) Hospital costs associated with surgical complications: a report from the private-sector National Surgical Quality Improvement Program. J Am Coll Surg 4(4):531–537
2. Chang AC, Yee J, Orringer MB, Iannettoni MD (2002) Diagnostic thoracoscopic lung biopsy: an outpatient experience. Ann Thorac Surg 74:1942–1947
3. Imai M (1986) Kaizen: the key to Japan's competitive success. Random House, New York

4. Iannettoni MD, Lynch WR, Parekh KR, McLaughlin KA (2011) Kaizen method for esophagectomy patients: improved quality control, outcomes, and decreased costs. Ann Thorac Surg 91(4):1011–1017
5. Katzenbach JR, Smith DK (2003) The wisdom of teams: creating the high-performance organization (Collins Business Essentials). Harper Paperbacks, New York

Perioperative Nutrition

14

Marco Braga

Surgery, like any injury to the body, elicits a series of reactions including release of stress hormones and inflammatory mediators. This release of mediators to the circulation has a major impact on body metabolism. It causes catabolism of glycogen, fat and protein with release of glucose, free fatty acids and amino acids into the circulation, so that substrates are in part diverted from the purposes they serve in the non-stressed state (i.e. physical activity) to the task of raising an adequate healing response. For optimal rehabilitation and wound healing, the body needs to be well nourished to mobilize adequate substrates, largely derived from muscle and adipose tissue, with nutritional support to allow synthesis of acute phase proteins, white cells, fibroblasts, collagen and other tissue components of the wounded area.

In modern surgical practice it is advisable to manage patients within an enhanced recovery protocol and thereby eating normal food within 2–4 days. However, the vast majority of patients with esophageal cancer undergoing surgery have suffered substantial weight loss, have very low body weight, i.e. body mass index (BMI) under 18.5–22 kg/m^2 depending on age, or exhibit inflammatory activity. Therefore, perioperative artificial nutrition should be considered almost routinely.

The main goals of perioperative nutritional support are to minimize negative protein balance by avoiding starvation, with the purpose to maintain muscle, immune, and cognitive function and to enhance postoperative recovery.

Energy substrates can be given either by the enteral or the parenteral route. Several studies have suggested a better outcome when at least part of the patient's requirement is met by the enteral route. There is some agreement that parenteral nutrition, when administered to patients who also tolerate enteral nutrition or who are not malnourished, causes more harm than benefit. In cases of prolonged postoperative gastrointestinal dysfunction, parenteral nutrition should be given until enteral function returns.

Traditionally, many patients undergoing esophageal resection used to receive large volumes of crystalloids intravenously during and after surgery. It was suggested that fluids and electrolytes were given in excess, resulting in substantial weight gain and edema. It was also suggested that this overload was a major cause of postoperative ileus and delayed gastric emptying. When fluids were restricted to the amount needed to maintain salt and water balance, gastro-intestinal function returned sooner and patients were capable of tolerating normal food and had bowel movements several days earlier than those in positive balance.

In recent years the traditional guidelines to fast patients overnight before elective surgery have been abandoned. The traditional routine was not based on solid evidence, while the evidence

M. Braga
Department of Surgery, San Raffaele University,
Via Olgettina 60, Milan 20132, Italy
e-mail: braga.marco@hsr.it

L. Bonavina (ed.), *Innovation in Esophageal Surgery*,
DOI 10.1007/978-88-470-2469-4_14, © Springer-Verlag Italia 2012

showing benefits and no harm when free intake of clear fluids was allowed until 2 h before anesthesia is substantially stronger. Consequently, many anesthesiology societies have changed their guidelines regarding fasting. This change in guidelines was prompted by the absence of evidence that fasting reduced the risks of aspiration. Allowing patients to drink also relieves the feeling of thirst that many patients experience before surgery.

14.1 Preoperative Nutrition

The influence of nutritional status on postoperative morbidity and mortality has been well documented in both retrospective and prospective studies. Two multivariate analyses have shown that undernutrition is an independent risk factor for the incidence of postoperative infectious complications, as well as increased mortality, length of hospital stay, and costs in patients undergoing curative surgery for upper gastrointestinal (GI) cancer.

Due to the risks associated with malnutrition and surgery, all patients undergoing esophageal surgery should be screened and assessed for nutritional status. The risk of severe undernutrition is considered by the European Society for Clinical Nutrition and Metabolism (ESPEN) working group to be present when at least one of the following criteria is present: weight loss >10–15 % within 6 months, BMI < 18 kg/m^2, Subjective Global Assessment: grade C, serum albumin <30 g/L (with no evidence of hepatic or renal dysfunction). On the basis of several reports in the literature, hypoalbuminemia reflects inflammatory activity and as such is a risk indicator of postoperative infectious complications and mortality rather than of the nutritional status itself [1, 2].

Several studies have demonstrated that 7–10 days of preoperative parenteral nutrition improve postoperative outcome in patients with severe undernutrition. However, preoperative parenteral nutrition is costly and can generally only be applied in the hospital setting by prolonging the length of stay [3].

Recently, the main focus of clinical nutrition has moved from the issue of energy and nitrogen requirement to the pharmacological effects of specific key nutrients. Standard nutritional feeds have been modified by adding specific substrates such as arginine, omega-3 fatty acids, and nucleotides. The main target of these new diets is not solely to provide energy and nitrogen, but to modulate inflammatory post-injury response and to counteract postoperative immune impairment which may *per se* increase patient susceptibility to infectious complications. Significant improvements in postoperative outcome have been reported using preoperative oral nutritional supplements enriched with specific immune-modulating substrates regardless of the baseline nutritional status. In fact, even well-nourished patients have been shown to develop an impaired immune response, an exuberant inflammatory response, and a reduction of splanchnic perfusion early after surgery. This approach is cheaper than parenteral nutrition and patients can be treated at home. It requires extra attention to ensure that oral supplements or nutritional drinks are actually taken by the patients.

In a recent meta-analysis Drover et al. [4] reviewed more than 30 random controlled trials (RCTs) including over 3,000 GI cancer patients undergoing elective surgery. Compared to a standard enteral formula, a diet supplemented with arginine and omega-3 fatty acids significantly reduced postoperative infectious complications and length of hospital stay also in the subgroup of upper GI cancer patients. These authors suggest that the supplementation of arginine and omega-3 fatty acids restores T-lymphocyte function including interleukin (IL)-2 production and also blunts the upregulation of immature myeloid-derived suppressor cells which usually occurs after major surgery.

It has been assumed that the traditional overnight fast preoperatively is useful and not harmful. However, over the last decade many national anesthesiology societies have changed preoperative fasting guidelines and now recommend free intake of clear fluids up until 2–3 h before anesthesia for elective procedures. This change has been proven safe and was brought about to reduce the discomfort of thirst. Allowing patients access to clear fluids up until 2 h prior to anesthesia also helps avoid preoperative dehydration. It has been recently shown that an iso-osmolar carbohydrate rich drink given preoperatively is quickly cleared from the stomach and, by the addition of carbohydrates, preoperative hunger and anxiety is also reduced. In addition and probably more important, by bringing the patient to surgery in a metabolically fed rather than fasted state, preoperative carbohydrate treatment reduces postoperative insulin resistance [5, 6].

The therapeutic goal for the postoperative patient is rapid recovery to normal function and well-being, the minimum of complications and early discharge home. This aim not only reflects good clinical practice but good economics. Minimising the development of catabolism and returning the patient from the catabolic state to one of anabolism is an important part of this process in which nutrition has a major role. Early oral intake and mobilization are the best weapons in this process.

14.2 Postoperative Parenteral Nutrition

Patients undergoing esophageal cancer surgery often exhibit nutritional depletion and run a higher risk of developing infectious complications. Postoperatively, oral intake is often delayed to protect the anastomosis or due to swelling, obstruction, impaired gastric emptying or paralytic ileus, making it difficult to meet nutritional requirements. In these patients surgeons should consider the placement of a feeding jejunostomy at the time of surgery. Daily nutritional targets are 25–27 kcal/kg and 1.5 g of protein/kg with an energy to nitrogen ratio of approximately 150:1.

Current guidelines recommend postoperative artificial nutrition for patients who cannot meet their caloric requirements within 3–5 days. In patients who require postoperative artificial nutrition, enteral feeding or a combination of enteral and supplementary parenteral feeding is the first choice. In fact, surgical patients fed enterally had an improved outcome compared with patients treated parenterally, and the nutrition-related sanitary costs are substantially reduced when the enteral route is used [7, 8].

In the case of prolonged gastrointestinal dysfunction, parenteral nutrition should be given until enteral function returns. In patients receiving parenteral nutrition, particular attention should be paid to avoiding too little or too much salt and water and to avoidance of hyperglycemia. For many of these patients, insulin may be needed to maintain glycemia between 110 and 150 mg/dL. Standard prescription can be used to give 30–40 % of total calories from fat [9].

When patients start taking oral food it is essential to monitor and record the adequacy of such intake. New anesthetic techniques for pain control, and the development of early postoperative recovery protocols allow the majority of patients to return to oral feeding very shortly after surgery. Consequently, the number of patients requiring postoperative nutritional support is progressively declining. For patients unable to consume sufficient amounts of food to meet basal needs, sip feeds can be recommended [10–12].

Nutritional care should be seen as an integral part of the optimal management of patients undergoing esophageal surgery and is no substitute for poor surgery or anesthesia or shortcomings in other aspects of care. Preoperative preparation, good surgery and anesthesia, optimal postoperative analgesia and fluid balance, and early mobilization and feeding form an integrated programme which in many centres is improving outcome and reducing hospital stay.

14.3 Standard Versus Personalized Nutrition

There are a number of situations in which standardized nutritional support cannot be applied:

- patients who suffer from heart failure may benefit from more concentrated nutrition, in which requirements are fulfilled in a lower volume. These patients sometimes require a sodium restricted regimen;
- patients with chronic renal failure and oliguria often require a restricted sodium and potassium regimen in low total volume. Protein/

nitrogen restriction is generally not recommended, because it may aggravate the malnutrition which is often accompanying chronic renal failure. The quality of renal replacement therapy has improved to such a degree that nitrogenous waste can efficiently be cleared even when liberal amounts of amino acids are included in the nutritional regimen;

- patients with hepatic failure have in the past been treated with low protein diets. This is obsolete. Very few patients will develop hepatic encephalopathy when receiving nutrition with normal amounts of protein. In fact, restriction induces a vicious circle by down-regulating enzymes in the urea cycle. Most patients therefore benefit from normal or even liberal amounts of protein/amino acids. In parenteral nutrition the induction of encephalopathy by amino acids in the nutritional mixture is even rarer and daily amounts up to 1.2–1.5 g of protein/kg ideal body weight may be safely administered. There is still some support for the claim that branched-chain amino acid (BCAA)-enriched parenteral nutrition is of benefit in liver patients and specifically those with impending or existing neurological signs.

Table 14.1 Daily requirements for vitamins in adults when given parenterally

Vitamin	Requirement
Thiamin (B1)	6 mg
Riboflavin (B2)	3.6 mg
Niacin (B3)	40 mg
Folic acid	600 mcg
Panthotenic acid	15 mg
Pyridoxine (B6)	6 mg
Cyanocobalamin (B12)	5 mcg
Biotin	60 mcg
Ascorbic Acid (C)	200 mg
Vitamin A	3,300 IU
Vitamin D	200 IU
Vitamin E	10 IU
Vitamin K	150 mcg

Table 14.2 Daily requirements for trace elements in adults when given parenterally

Trace element	Requirement
Chromium	10–15 mcg
Copper	0.3–0.5 mg
Iron	1.0–1.2 mg
Manganese	50–100 mcg
Selenium	60–100 mcg
Zinc	2.5–5 mg
Molybdenum	20 mcg
Iodine	130 mcg
Fluoride	1 mg

14.4 Vitamins and Trace Elements

In wellnourished patients who recover oral or enteral nutrition within postoperative day 4 there is little evidence that intravenous supplementation of vitamins and trace elements is required. In those patients who are unable to be fed via the enteral route after surgery and in whom total or near total parenteral nutrition is required, a full range of vitamins and trace elements should be supplemented on a daily basis.

When early oral food intake/enteral nutrition is combined with parenteral nutrition, intravenous supplementation of vitamins appears to be unnecessary. In the case of total parenteral nutrition, a consensus exists that micronutrients/antioxidants should be supplemented on a daily basis. In accordance with the US Food and Drug Administration the recommendations for vitamins provision were recently updated (Table 14.1).

The daily requirements for trace elements in surgical patients are more variable, due to the potential depletion on commencing artificial nutrition, the effects of surgery, and concerns regarding liver or kidney dysfunction. Recommendations provided in Table 14.2 are therefore for a typical surgical patient, without increased gut losses, and with normal liver and kidney function. They are based upon American Society for Parenteral and Enteral Nutrition (ASPEN) recommendations from 2004, but modified at the 2009 ASPEN Research Workshop (unpublished data). Zinc requirement in particular will be increased if there are high fluid losses from the gut [13, 14].

Key Points

- Adequate perioperative nutritional support is critical to maintain muscle, immune, and cognitive function, and to enhance postoperative recovery in esophageal surgery
- The focus of clinical nutrition has moved from the issue of energy and nitrogen requirement to the pharmacological effects of specific key nutrients such as arginine, omega-3 fatty acids, and nucleotides
- The target of this new nutritional approach is to modulate inflammatory post-injury response and to counteract postoperative immune impairment which may *per se* increase patient susceptibility to infectious complications

References

1. Weimann A, Braga M, Harsanyi L, Laviano A, Ljungqvist O, Soeters P (2006) ESPEN guidelines on enteral nutrition: surgery including organ transplantation. Clin Nutr 25:224–244
2. Braga M, Ljungqvist O, Soeters P, Fearon KC, Bozzetti F (2009) ESPEN guidelines on parenteral nutrition in surgery. Clin Nutr 28:378–386
3. Kehlet H (1997) Multimodal approach to control postoperative pathophysiology and rehabilitation. Br J Anaesth 78:606–617
4. Drover JW, Dhaliwal R, Weitzel L et al (2011) Perioperative use of arginine-supplemented diets: a systematic review of the evidence. J Am Coll Surg 212:385–399
5. Ljungqvist O, Soreide E (2003) Preoperative fasting. Br J Surg 90:400–406
6. Lassen K, Kjeve J, Fetveit T et al (2008) Allowing normal food at will after major upper gastrointestinal surgery does not increase morbidity. A randomized multicenter Trial. Ann Surg 247:721–729
7. Braga M, Gianotti L, Gentilini O, Parisi V, Salis C, Di Carlo V (2001) Early postoperative enteral nutrition improves gut oxygenation and reduces costs compared with total parenteral nutrition. Crit Care Med 29:242–248
8. Bozzetti F, Braga M, Gianotti L, Gavazzi C, Mariani L (2001) Postoperative enteral versus parenteral nutrition in malnourished patients with gastrointestinal cancer: a randomised multicentre trial. Lancet 358: 1487–1492
9. Lobo DN, Bostock KA, Neal KR, Perkins AC, Rowlands BJ, Allison SP (2002) Effect of salt and water balance on recovery of gastrointestinal function after elective colonic resection: a randomised controlled trial. Lancet 359:1812–1818
10. (1991) Perioperative total parenteral nutrition in surgical patients. The Veterans Affairs Total Parenteral Nutrition Cooperative Study Group. N Engl J Med 325:525–532
11. Heyland DK, Montalvo M, MacDonald S et al (2001) Total parenteral nutrition in the surgical patient: a meta-analysis. Can J Surg 44:102–111
12. Mirtallo J, Canada T, Johnson D, Kumpf V, Petersen C, Sacks G, Seres D, Guenter P, Task Force for the Revision of Safe Practices for Parenteral Nutrition (2004) Safe practices for parenteral nutrition. J Parenter Enteral Nutr 29:S39–S70
13. Berger MM, Shenkin A (2006) Vitamins and trace elements: practical aspects of supplementation. Nutrition 22:952–955
14. Food and Drug Administration (FDA) (2000) Parenteral multivitamin products; drugs for human use; drug efficacy study implementation; amendment. Fed Regist 65:21200–21201

Quality Assessment, Education and Training in Esophageal Surgery

15

Arnulf H. Hölscher and Ulrich K. Fetzner

15.1 Quality Assessment

In general, quality assessment concerns structure of the institution, management processes and results. The structural components of the institution are not the focus of this chapter, but rather the surgical management and results.

Indicators and outcome measurements for esophageal surgery have to be differentiated concerning the preoperative, intraoperative or postoperative phase. For the latter, short-term and long-term results are usually reported.

15.1.1 Preoperative

Preoperative quality assessment in patients with malignant diseases of the esophagus or the esophagogastric junction comprises:

- the exact localization and extent of the carcinoma;
- the clinical tumor, node, metastasis (TNM) staging; and
- the detailed evaluation of the functional risk.

All these issues are important to choose the adequate individualized therapy [1]. Therefore, the quality of endoscopy, histology and abdominal or thoracic computed tomography (CT)-scan have a special significance. Clinical TNM staging, histology, size and extent of the tumor are the basis for decision about the therapeutic spectrum which ranges from endoscopic removal to primary surgery or neoadjuvant radio-chemotherapy followed by surgical resection [2, 3] (Fig. 15.1) and (Fig. 15.2).

In the case of induction therapy, the quality of neoadjuvant chemotherapy or chemoradiation is of special influence on the short- and long-term surgical results [4, 5]. The quality of selection of treatment has enormous consequences on the therapeutic short- and long-term results. Further, assessment of the functional risk of the individual patient is very important to avoid intra- or postoperative complications by prophylactic measures as well as to aid the awareness of the therapeutic team. We advocate a detailed preoperative risk analysis with a score differentiating normal, medium and high risk [6]. On the basis of this analysis the postoperative course and postoperative mortality can be predicted.

A.H. Hölscher, M.D. (✉) • U.K. Fetzner
Department of General,
Visceral and Cancer Surgery,
University of Cologne, Cologne, Germany
e-mail: arnulf.hoelscher@uk-koeln.de

L. Bonavina (ed.), *Innovation in Esophageal Surgery*,
DOI 10.1007/978-88-470-2469-4_15, © Springer-Verlag Italia 2012

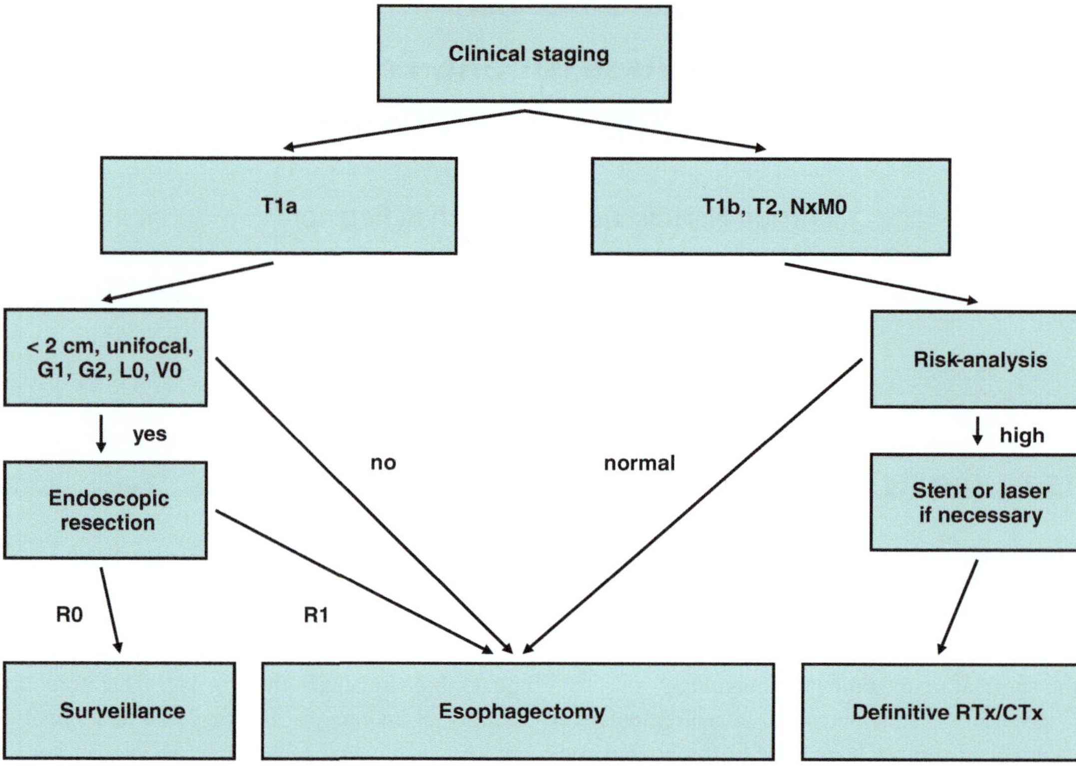

Fig. 15.1 Algorithm for treatment strategy in T1 or T2 esophageal carcinoma (Modified from [7])

In benign functional diseases of the esophagus, the exact diagnosis and the quantitative evaluation of its severity are of great importance for the therapeutic decisions [7]. Examples are manometry or impedance measurement for achalasia and esophageal pH-monitoring for reflux disease. If the diagnosis is not exact the choice of therapy may be wrong with severe consequences on short- or long-term outcome.

15.1.2 Intraoperative

The experience of the surgeon and of the whole team including anesthesiologists, pathologists for frozen section and scrub nurses is important for the result of the operation. Measurable indicators of intraoperative surgical quality in general are:

- number of blood transfusions;
- duration of operation;and for malignant diseases:
- resection without residual disease (R0-resection) [8]; and
- number of resected lymph nodes [3].

As an example, allogeneic blood transfusion not only has an influence on the short-term postoperative outcome but also on long-term survival in patients with esophageal cancer. We showed that patients with transfusion of 0–1 units of blood have a significantly better long-term prognosis compared to those patients with transfusion of more than 1 unit of blood [9].

15.1.3 Postoperative

15.1.3.1 Short-Term Results

The short-term results are especially dependent on the experience of the surgeon, the nursing team and, in the case of major surgery, on the experience of the intensive care unit (ICU) team.

Indicators of quality are:

- postoperative complications;
- percentage of reoperations;
- postoperative mortality;
- days in ICU;
- days in hospital.

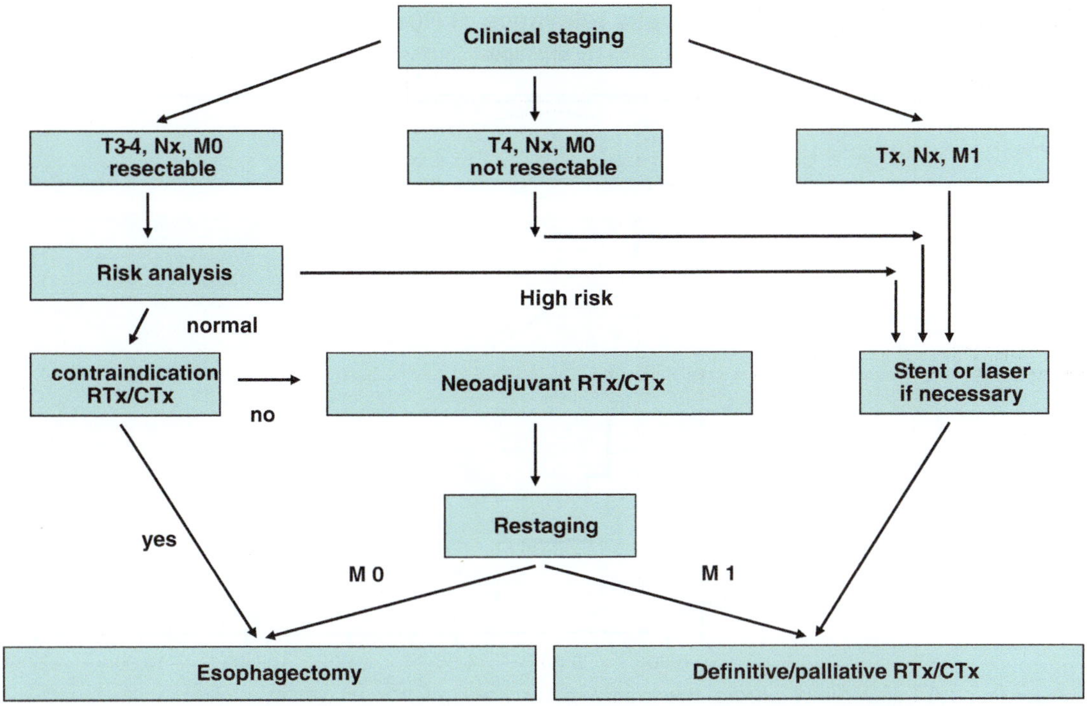

Fig. 15.2 Algorithm for treatment strategy in T3 or T4 esophageal carcinoma (Modified from [7])

The main postoperative complications in esophageal cancer surgery are pneumonia and anastomotic leak. In a recent analysis of 858 patients undergoing esophagectomy for cancer, pulmonary complications were reported in 27.4 % and anastomotic insufficiency in 12.5 % [10]. Postoperative complications also have an influence on long-term survival [11]. Therefore, avoidance of postoperative morbidity is not only meaningful for the immediate benefit it brings but also in the long run.

The most important indicator, however, is postoperative mortality. Recent results of major centers of esophageal surgery show a postoperative fatal outcome in less than 5 % (Table 15.1). This can be considered as the current standard. It is interesting that neither the frequency of anastomotic leak (12.2 vs. 12.5 %) nor mortality (3.5 vs. 3.5 %) were different comparing open (n=394) to minimally invasive (n=464) esophagectomy [10].

15.1.3.2 Long-Term Results

The quality indicators of long-term outcome after esophagectomy for cancer are:

Table 15.1 Compilation of the results of postoperative mortality in esophageal cancer surgery [10–13]

Author	Time span	Patients	Mortality (%)
Mariette et al. [13]	1994–2002	536	5.0
Lerut et al. [11]	2005–2006	138	1.4
Schröder et al. [12]	2003–2010	419	4.3
Zingg et al. [10]	1989–2008	858	3.5

- disease free survival;
- overall survival;
- symptoms;
- body weight;
- quality of life.

As an example, the influence of R0 resection on long-term survival in 243 patients with esophagectomy for cancer is shown in Fig. 15.3. Further, the number of the resected lymph nodes is important for long-term survival [14]. This is not only true for patients with lymph node metastasis but also for those in the pN0 category which includes those with micrometastasis that are not detected on routine histopathologic work up [15].

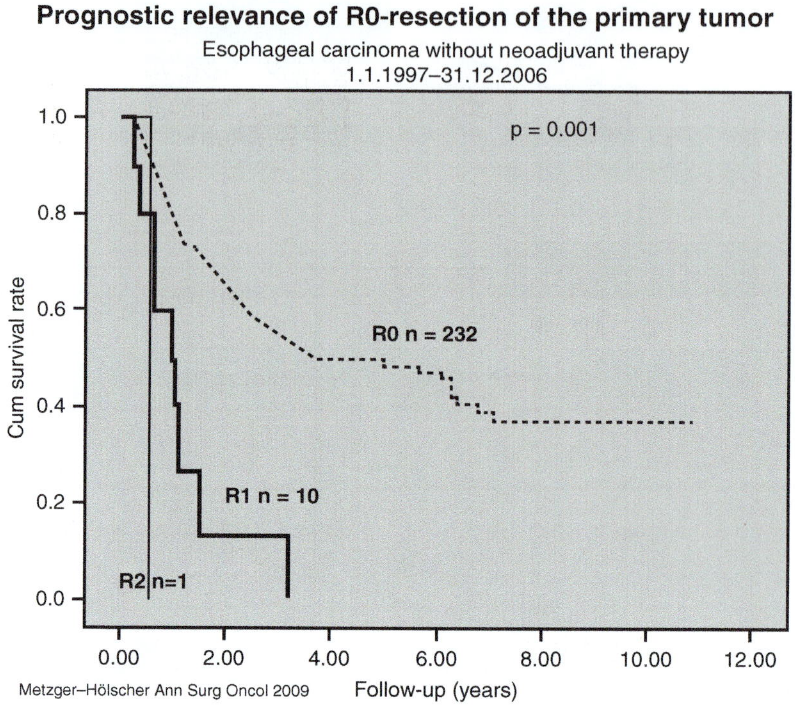

Fig. 15.3 Prognostic relevance of R0 resection in 243 own patients with esophagectomy for cancer without neoadjuvant therapy (From [8])

Symptoms like swallowing disorders, body weight and quality of life are important outcome parameters in patients with malignant as well as benign diseases of the esophagus that are treated by surgery. The reoperation rate in the long term can be an indicator of surgical quality in gastroesophageal reflux disease.

Many papers have shown that patients undergoing esophagectomy for cancer have a better short-term and long-term outcome after surgery in high volume centers than in low volume institutions [16, 17]. The annual number of esophagectomies per year is an indirect surrogate parameter that is inferior to direct outcome criteria. However, volume is a quite reproducible indicator for quality, especially concerning mortality. In order to improve the results after esophagectomy, several countries like Great Britain and Germany have concentrated the performance of esophageal surgery in larger institutions. The first results are promising [18].

15.2 Education and Training

Both, the decathlete and the esophageal surgeon need:

- skillfulness;
- universalism; and
- power of endurance.

Day 1 and day 2 in a decathlon are comparable to the two-cavity operation in abdomen and chest in esophageal surgery. The esophageal surgeon like the decathlete needs knowledge and skillfulness in different disciplines. This is because the esophagus crosses different regions: the neck, the chest and the abdomen. The esophagus can develop malignant and benign diseases. The esophagus affords various kinds of diagnostics. The therapeutic options comprise operation, interventional procedures and medication. The surgical techniques nowadays are performed with an open or a minimally invasive approach. Most patients with esophageal cancer have multiple

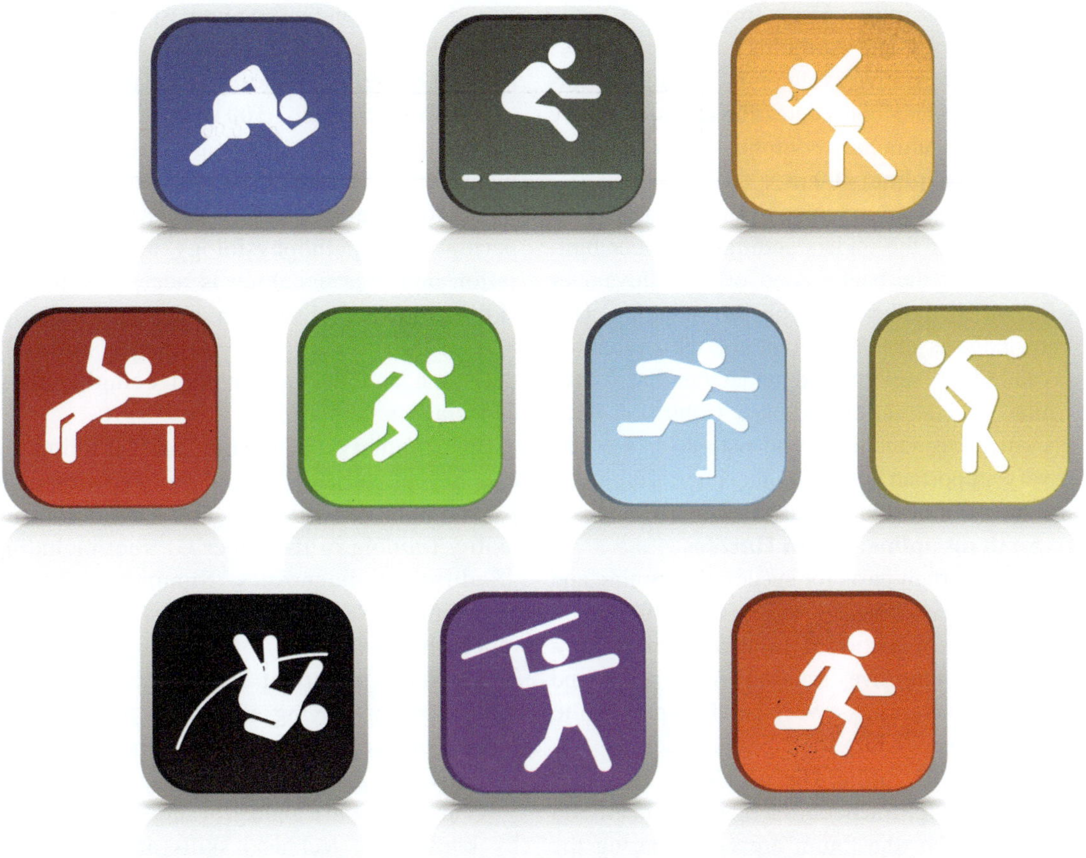

Fig. 15.4 Decathlon disciplines

comorbidities. In many patients extensive surgery is performed and intensive care has a profound impact on the final outcome.

The following ten disciplines which are important for education and training of the esophageal surgeon are compared to a decathlon (Fig. 15.4).

First discipline: 100 m

The etiology of diseases, the anatomy, the esophageal physiology and pathophysiology represent the basic knowledge that is necessary to understand esophageal problems and decide about therapeutic choices. Representative for esophageal physiology are pH-monitoring, manometry and impedance measurement.

Second discipline: Long Jump

Endoscopy and endosonography are very important diagnostic tools for surveillance of patients with esophageal diseases, for primary staging of cancer, for evaluation of benign diseases, for detection of postoperative complications and for endoscopic follow up.

Third discipline: Shot put

Radiology and nuclear medicine comprising CT scan of abdomen and thorax, magnetic resonance imaging (MRI), positron emission tomography (PET), CT and ultrasound are important tools for primary staging of cancer, for evaluation of resectability, for evaluation of functional diseases and detection of postoperative complications.

Fourth discipline: High Jump

Pneumology and cardiology are very important for preoperative evaluation of lung and cardiac function and for the detection of postoperative cardiac and pulmonary complications.

Fifth discipline: 400 m

Knowledge in oncology and pathology is necessary for the understanding of cancer biology and for the background of neoadjuvant or adjuvant chemotherapy or chemo-radiation. This knowledge is also important for the evaluation of pathology reports and understanding of the Union for International Cancer Control (UICC) classification. Oncology and pathology are also a very important basis for the interdisciplinary management of esophageal cancer.

Sixth discipline: 110 m Hurdles

An important basis for successful training and education in esophageal surgery is skillfulness in general and in particular in abdominal surgery. Therefore, intensive training in general and abdominal surgery is a very good preparation to become a successful esophageal surgeon.

Seventh discipline: Discus Throw

As the lung, tracheobronchial tree, heart and aorta in the mediastinum are neighbouring the esophagus, knowledge in the field of thoracic and vascular surgery is very important for the performance of primary surgery and for treating complications of surgery.

Eighth discipline: Pole Vault

Neck surgery is an important part of the education for an esophageal surgeon. The special anatomy of the neck, the course of the recurrent laryngeal nerve, and the anatomy and function of the hypopharynx, larynx and upper esophageal sphincter are very important issues for the esophageal surgeon.

Ninth discipline: Javelin Throw

Minimally invasive surgery has become an important part of esophageal operations. It embraces thoracic as well as abdominal surgery. An open mind and a keen interest in new technical devices is a good prerequisite for continuous medical education of the esophageal surgeon.

Tenth discipline: 1,500 m

Finally, the intensive care unit is an area where many things in the postoperative phase come to a culmination point. Knowledge of perioperative pathophysiology, artificial respiration and pharmacology is necessary for the skilled esophageal surgeon. Further, the esophageal surgeon has to be informed about early detection and management of complications, especially sepsis.

In summary, education and training in esophageal surgery should be performed as part of both general surgical training and speciality training of the upper GI tract including all different diagnostics. Simulation courses for minimally invasive surgery support very much the skillfulness of the esophageal surgeon. Many important surgeons have had the advantage of having the right mentor who taught, criticized and corrected them and who was always open for questions.

Competence in esophageal surgery is achieved by knowledge, technical skills and behaviour. Both the decathlete and the esophageal surgeon must be skillful, sustained and all-round. The decathlete is the athletic king. Is the esophageal surgeon the king of surgery?

Key Points

- Esophageal surgery is by definition a true multidisciplinary field
- The esophageal surgeon, like the decathlete, needs knowledge and skillfulness in different disciplines
- Center volume is a quite reproducible indicator for quality in esophageal surgery

References

1. Hölscher AH (2008) Adenocarcinoma of the cardia. In: Pearson F (ed) Pearson's thoracic and esophageal surgery, 3rd edn. Churchill Livingstone/Elsevier, Philadelphia, pp 492–497
2. Hölscher AH, Bollschweiler E, Schröder W, Metzger R, Gutschow C, Drebber U (2011) Prognostic impact of upper, middle, and lower third mucosal or submucosal infiltration in early esophageal cancer. Ann Surg 254:802–807; discussion 807–808
3. Hölscher AH, Lordick F (2012) Chirurgische und internistische Diagnostik und Therapie des Ösophaguskarzinoms. Gastroenterologie up2date 8 2012, Thieme publisher Stuttgart
4. Schneider P, Baldus S, Metzger R, Kocher M, Bongartz R, Bollschweiler E, Schaefer H, Thiele J, Dienes H, Müller R, Hölscher A (2005) Histomorphologic tumor regression and lymph node metastases determine prognosis following neoadjuvant radiochemotherapy for esophageal cancer: implications for response classification. Ann Surg 242:684–692
5. Vallböhmer D, Hölscher AH, Dietlein M et al (2009) [18F]-Fluorodeoxyglucose-positron emission tomography for the assessment of histopathologic response and prognosis after completion of neoadjuvant chemoradiation in esophageal cancer. Ann Surg 250:888–894
6. Schröder W, Bollschweiler E, Kossow C, Hölscher A (2006) Preoperative risk analysis – a reliable predictor of postoperative outcome after transthoracic esophagectomy? Langenbecks Arch Surg 391:455–460
7. Hölscher AH (2006) Ösophagus. In: Becker H, Encke A, Röher HD (eds) Viszeralchirurgie, 2nd edn. Urban & Fischer, München/Jena, pp 369–410
8. Metzger R, Drebber U, Baldus SE, Mönig SP, Hölscher AH, Bollschweiler E (2009) Extracapsular lymph node involvement differs between squamous cell and adenocarcinoma of the esophagus. Ann Surg Oncol 16:447–453
9. Ling F, Hölscher A, Vallböhmer D, Schmidt D, Picker S, Gathof B, Bollschweiler E, Schneider P (2009) Leukocyte depletion in allogeneic blood transfusion does not change the negative influence on survival following transthoracic resection for esophageal cancer. J Gastrointest Surg 13:581–586
10. Zingg U, Smithers BM, Gotley DC, Smith G, Aly A, Clough A, Esterman AJ, Jamieson GG, Watson DI (2011) Factors associated with postoperative pulmonary morbidity after esophagectomy for cancer. Ann Surg Oncol 18:1460–1468
11. Lerut T, Moons J, Coosemans W, Van Raemdonck D, De Leyn P, Decaluwe H, Decker G, Nafteux P (2009) Postoperative complications after transthoracic esophagectomy for cancer of the esophagus and gastroesophageal junction are correlated with early cancer recurrence: role of systematic grading of complications using the modified Clavien classification. Ann Surg 250:798–807
12. Schröder W, Hölscher AH, Bludau M, Vallböhmer D, Bollschweiler E, Gutschow C (2010) Ivor-lewis esophagectomy with and without laparoscopic conditioning of the gastric conduit. World J Surg 34: 738–743
13. Mariette C, Piessen G, Briez N, Triboulet JP (2008) The number of metastatic lymph nodes and the ratio between metastatic and examined lymph nodes are independent prognostic factors in esophageal cancer regardless of neoadjuvant chemoradiation or lymphadenectomy extent. Ann Surg 247: 365–371
14. Peyre C, Hagen J, De Meester S, Altorki N, Ancona E, Griffin S, Hölscher A, Lerut T, Law S, Rice T, Ruol A, van Lanschot J, Wong J, De Meester T (2008) The number of lymph nodes removed predicts survival in esophageal cancer: an international study on the impact of extent of surgical resection. Ann Surg 248:549–556
15. Bollschweiler E, Baldus S, Schröder W, Schneider P, Hölscher A (2006) Staging of esophageal carcinoma: length of tumor and number of involved regional lymph nodes. Are these independent prognostic factors? J Surg Oncol 94:355–363
16. Metzger R, Bollschweiler E, Vallböhmer D, Maish M, De Meester T, Hölscher A (2004) High volume centers for esophagectomy: what is the number needed to achieve low postoperative mortality? Dis Esophagus 17:310–314
17. Rouvelas I, Jia C, Viklund P, Lindblad M, Lagergren J (2007) Surgeon volume and postoperative mortality after oesophagectomy for cancer. Eur J Surg Oncol 33:162–168
18. Al-Sarira A, David G, Willmott S, Slavin J, Deakin M, Corless D (2007) Oesophagectomy practice and outcomes in England. Br J Surg 94:585–591

The Future of Esophageal Surgery 16

Tom R. DeMeester

Not long ago before a New York audience of general surgeons I was asked the question: what will be the future of esophageal surgery? My answer, based on personal sagacity, conjecture and guesses, was designed not to speculate what is to be, but to stimulate what could be. In short, I said General Surgery will be forced into sub-specialization and esophageal will become part of a subspecialty called Foregut Surgery. The reason for my prediction was the existence of strong forces that are pushing general surgery in this direction. The movement towards sub-specialization is a natural phenomenon. Stones drop, water wets, fire burns and knowledge begets sub-specialization. Resistance to this natural process can slow it down, but can never stop the inevitable flow from reaching its natural end. The working schema of this natural process is: new knowledge fosters specialization, specialization fosters new technology, and new technology fosters new knowledge. By this process the present becomes history and the future labeled progress. This phenomenon caused a movement away from traditional open surgery to laparoscopic surgery and from laparoscopic surgery to endoscopic endo-luminal and trans-luminal surgery. The most recent example of this process is the introduction of the POEM procedure (Per Oral Endoscopic Myotomy) for achalasia [1]. A consequence of this natural phenomenon has been a 60 % reduction in open general surgical case volume [2].

T.R. DeMeester
Department of Surgery, Keck School of Medicine, University of Southern California, Los Angeles, CA, USA
e-mail: tdemeester@surgery.usc.edu

Another force pushing sub-specialization is the current state of surgical therapy in the United States. There are ten million general surgical operations performed each year in the United States at a cost of one billion US dollars. The overall operative mortality is 2 % and the complication rate is 13 %. Two-thirds of the mortalities and complications are due to intra-operative errors. Sixty-four percent of the intra-operative errors are technical and 29 % are errors of judgment, and both are due to a lack of experience [3–6]. The operative mortality of complicated surgical procedures such as esophageal, pancreatic, and liver resections is high when performed by inexperienced surgeons in low numbers in poorly equipped and inadequately staffed hospitals. In contrast, the operative mortality and complication rate is lower when these operations are performed by adequately trained surgeons, on large numbers of patients, in properly equipped and staffed hospitals [7–10]. Together these studies give rise to the hypothesis that specifically trained surgeons, with a narrow clinical focus and working in properly equipped and staffed hospitals, would reduce the operative mortality and the rate of surgical complications in the U.S.

A third force pushing sub-specialization is the market place. To illustrate this I ask the reader to pick out the misfit in the following fields of surgery: General Surgery, Ophthalmology, Otorhinolaryngology, Orthopedic Surgery, Urology

L. Bonavina (ed.), *Innovation in Esophageal Surgery*,
DOI 10.1007/978-88-470-2469-4_16, © Springer-Verlag Italia 2012

and Vascular Surgery. If you picked out General Surgery you were correct. The term General Surgery is the only term of the six that does not describe the focus of its livelihood. Consequently, it does not have a direct link to patients. Further, General Surgery is unique as the only field of surgery that does not provide a diagnostic service. Consequently, it is perceived by patients to be only of therapeutic benefit. In a world of specific surgical options the term General Surgery is too broad and nondescript to have an effect in today's health care market place. Esophageal surgery, as long as it is buried within General Surgery, will be stifled in providing a full diagnostic, endoscopic and therapeutic service to patients. In contrast, the growth in Colorectal Surgery is largely due to its status as an independent subspecialty and the specific training of the involved surgeons in a narrow clinical focus with both a diagnostic and therapeutic emphasis.

The strongest force pushing sub-specialization is the status of resident training in General Surgery. Directors of General Surgery residency programs in the United States were requested to review a list of >300 types of surgical procedures that made up the case-log used by residents to document their training experience. They were instructed to identify those "essential" procedures a general surgical resident should be competent to perform prior to obtaining permission to practice. From the list, they identified 121 procedures thought to be "essential" to general surgery practice. The summited resident case-logs were then reviewed. As would be expected, the most common "essential" operation reported was laparoscopic cholecystectomy. The most common number of operations done in 52 % of the identified 121 "essential" operations was 0 and included common bile duct exploration, transanal tumor excision and anorectal fistula [2]. More telling is a statement by Dr. Frank Lewis, Executive Director of the American Board of Surgery. He stated that the surgical experience of a General Surgical resident during their chief year of residency has dropped from 400 to 500 operations per year to 150. Minimally invasive procedures accounted for 60 % of the 150 operations. According to Dr. Lewis most residents are uncomfortable with open procedures and seek additional training after residency in focused subspecialty fellowships [11]. Dr. K. Anders Ericsson, a cognitive Psychologist, stated that "it takes > 10,000 hours of practice for a person to develop 'expertise' in a complex task" [12]. This number equals approximately 8 h/day of deliberate practice for 5 years. The hours residents spend doing "essential" operations during 5 years of residency is only 1,148 [13]. The field of General Surgery is just too broad to expect the resident to master the knowledge and practical skill necessary to become competent in all of the procedures that make up the field. Training in General Surgery needs to become narrower with a focus on one of the sub-specialties emerging in the field.

Pressure from patients is also pushing subspecialization. Patients focus on their disease, not surgery. Consequently they seek out consultation and guidance from physicians who are identified with their disease. Surgery is the farthest from the patients mind and, if at all possible, something to be avoided. Surgeons are rarely sought out by patients and consultants in other fields rarely discuss the option of surgical therapy even when indicated. If the topic of referral for surgical therapy should come up at all, the patient is usually referred to a surgeon who focuses on the specific organ system that the disease involves. Further, if a surgical therapy becomes less invasive, one of the focused nonsurgical specialties will learn the less invasive technique and perform it. In this way the surgical disciplines, particularly general surgeons, are bypassed unless they have developed a specific reputation in a focused organ system that is both diagnostic and therapeutic. Failure of General Surgery to sub-specialize into focused fields and develop a diagnostic arm is devaluating General Surgery to the level of a procedural craft with minimal diagnostic and scientific value.

To correct the current state of General Surgery and allow esophageal surgery to flourish will require that General Surgery undergo a reformation without deformation. Surgery must be redefined, its public image improved, its diagnostic and endoscopic capacities fostered and the field reorganized into focused sub-specialties.

Diagnostic laboratories must emerge in each subspecialty to test for and define the degree of pathophysiology in the diseased organs surgeon treat. Dr. Atul Gawande has astutely stated that the focus of surgery has shifted "over time from a specialty defined by 'manual operation' to one defined by concern with the diseases that might need an operation. This is ... a crucial difference. For it is the difference between whether we aim to create technicians or aim to create doctors" [13]. In other words, surgery is changing from a technical act to a unique form of therapy. A therapy is motivated by compassion, applied cognitively by an informed and experienced mind using measured indications, planned and rehearsed in an educated brain and executed by hands trained to deliver the therapy in the most minimally invasive manner.

Of interest, surgeons can perform endoscopy in Canada, Germany, Austria and Italy. In United States surgeons in rural areas can perform endoscopy but in metropolitan areas, due to opposition from local gastroenterologists, the privilege is restricted to various degrees. In France surgeons are forbidden to do endoscopy. For a surgeon to regain endoscopic privileges when they have been lost can be difficult. It can commonly lead to confrontation and interrogation by gastroenterologists. The surgeon is often questioned regarding their knowledge of endoscopy, the indication for the procedure, the use of conscious sedation and the various techniques in performing endoscopy. The interrogation is the battle front and surgeons need to prepare for it. They must know the endoscopic literature and be ready to site chapter and verse in answering the questions asked. The end of the challenge will be signaled when a gastroenterologist, unexpectedly, describes how and when the surgeon would perform an endoscopic procedure on one of their patients and asks the surgeon to affirm his description.. If the surgeon acknowledges it to be correct, the gastroenterologist is likely to refer the patient to the surgeon to do what he, the gastroenterologist stated the surgeon would do. This not uncommon initial ritual will mark the point of transition from resistance to acceptance of the surgeon as an endoscopist. This transition point will indicate that the surgeon is respected for his knowledge, skill and value in the management of patients with complex gastrointestinal abnormalities.

To reform General Surgery requires breaking it down into well thought through sub-specialties, each with its own focused area of interest and educational objectives. A list of such sub-specialties are : (1) Foregut Diseases, (2) Hepato-pancreatico-billary Diseases, (3) Colorectal Diseases, (4) Breast, soft tissue tumors and Endocrine Diseases, (5) Trauma and acute care surgery, (6) Rural surgical care, and (7) Surgical intensive care. Under this scenario the sub-specialty of Foregut Diseases would include the diagnosis and surgical therapy of diseases of the pharynx, esophagus, gastroesophageal junction, stomach, duodenum and small bowel down to the jejuno-ileo junction. The option exists that this could also include bariatric surgery. Surgeons interested in this subspecialty would acquire the knowledge and skills to diagnose the various foregut abnormalities and perform open, laparoscopic and endoscopic surgical procedures to treat the diseases when appropriate.

To obtain the knowledge and skill specific to each sub-specialty will require a restructuring of the General Surgery residency. In years 1 and 2 the residents would focus on learning the day to day care of surgical patients, bedside operative procedures and minor surgical procedures in the operating room. A future goal would be to begin the 1st year of residency in the 4th year of medical school with the possibly of adding a 5th year to the medical school curriculum to accommodate the 2nd year of residency. In years 3, 4, and 5 the residents would begin their sub-specialty training in both diagnostic and therapeutic procedures. For example, in the subspecialty of Foregut Surgery this would include upper gastrointestinal endoscopy, endoscopic ultrasound, esophageal motility, ambulatory esophageal and gastric pH monitoring, interpreting of upper gastrointestinal radiological contrast studies reading, CT or MRI imaging studies and the endoscopic, laparoscopic and open surgical procedures used to treat foregut diseases.

Consideration should be given to organizing the delivery of surgical care by the sub-specialties of General Surgery in a manner similar to the proposed Accountable Care Organization (ACO) in the current U. S. Affordable Care Act. ACOs are primary care provider-based organizations that take responsibility for meeting the health care needs of a defined population with the goal of simultaneously improving health, improving patient experience, and reducing per capita costs. An organization similar to an ACO could be designed to provide a delivery vehicle for surgical sub-specialty care. I would call this modified ACO an Accountable Care Center (ACC). ACCs would be provider-based centers of excellence that take responsibility for the diagnosis, treatment, and follow-up of patients with specific high volume diseases involving a specific organ system with the goal of simultaneously improving the care, improving patient experience, and reducing the overall per capita costs of managing diseases of a specific organ system. This proposed method of health care delivery requires that the various surgical sub-specialties develop ACCs around high volume diseases in their focused area of interest in independent out-patient centers. Since a high volume disease of a specific organ system usually accounts for 80 % of the work load of a subspecialty, ACCs should be able to take on the responsibility to reduce the per capita cost for all the diseases involving their specific organ system. They would maximize screening and surveillance, provide efficient and accurate out-patient diagnostic testing, correctly determining when surgical therapy is indicated, perform efficient, safe and effective outpatient surgical therapy and have aligned relationships with hospitals for the cost effective care for patients that need inpatient services or operations. The medical staff of an ACC would consist of multidisciplinary physicians, all with a focused interest in the same organ system. In such a center the majority of medical and surgical care for esophageal disease could be provided in an outpatient setting at considerable less expense. Once established, the ACC would be incentivized to reduce cost of care through innovative non-surgical treatment strategies and less invasive outpatient surgical procedures. Physicians and surgeons hold the future of health care reform in their hands. Ultimately, the success or failure of change in the health-care system hinges largely on them. The organization of an ACC is one way physicians and surgeons can co-operate to provide innovative low cost, high quality and efficient care of patients with diseases of a specific organ system. The side benefits of such an approach is a strong incentive to detect disease at an earlier stage and a more efficient care of patients with advanced disease.

To reform surgery in such a manner need not deform a clinical science that has made many spectacular contributions to the wellbeing of humanity. To preserve surgery while shaping it for the future will require the type of leadership that brings surgeons out of isolation into community and to orchestrate a rebuilding of surgery in a manner they cannot do as a surgeon alone. Tomorrow's surgical leaders must have the gift to integrate and combine the not yet combined and integrated. Surgeons must become both individual and institutional minded: without individuals nothing happens, without institutions nothing survives.

Key Points

- General Surgery is being forced progressively into sub-specialization and esophageal surgery is likely to become part of a subspecialty called Foregut Surgery
- Well trained surgeons, with a narrow clinical focus on specific organ systems and working in properly equipped and staffed hospitals, will be expected to provide safer, less expensive and better surgical therapy in the future
- Patients focus on their disease and seek out consultation and guidance from surgeons who master one domain of knowledge and are expert in specific diagnostic and therapeutic procedures
- The General Surgery sub-specialties should develop both a diagnostic and therapeutic arm of patient management
- General Surgery needs to explore new models for the delivery of surgical therapy that fit with the changing demands of health care

References

1. Inoue H, Minami H, Kobayashi Y et al (2010) Peroral endoscopic myotomy (POEM) for esophageal achalasia. Endoscopy 265(42):265–271
2. Bell RH Jr, Biester TW, Tabuenca A et al (2009) Operative experience of residents in US general surgery programs: a gap between expectation and experience. Ann Surg 249:719–724
3. Ritchie WP Jr, Rhodes RS, Biester TW (1999) Work loads and practice patterns of general surgeons in the United States, 1995–1997: a report from the American Board of Surgery. Ann Surg 230:533–543
4. Khuri SF, Henderson WG, Daley J et al (2008) Successful implementation of the Department of Veterans Affairs' National Surgical Quality Improvement Program in the private sector: the Patient Safety in Surgery study. Ann Surg 248:329–336
5. Gawande AA, Zinner MJ, Studdert DM, Brennan TA (2003) Analysis of errors reported by surgeons at three teaching hospitals. Surgery 133:614–621
6. Fabri PJ, Zayas-Castro JL (2008) Human error, not communication and systems, underlies surgical complications. Surgery 144:557–563
7. Dimick JB, Goodney PP, Orringer MB, Birkmeyer JD (2005) Specialty training and mortality after esophageal cancer resection. Ann Thorac Surg 80:282–286
8. Dimick JB, Birkmeyer JD, Upchurch GR Jr (2005) Measuring surgical quality: what's the role of provider volume? World J Surg 29:1217–1221
9. Birkmeyer JD, Siewers AE, Finlayson EV et al (2002) Hospital volume and surgical mortality in the United States. N Engl J Med 346:1128–1137
10. Begg CB, Cramer LD, Hoskins WJ, Brennan MF (1998) Impact of hospital volume on operative mortality for major cancer surgery. JAMA 280:1747–1751
11. Oral report given by Dr. Frank Lewis, Executive Director of the American Board of Surgery, to the 2011 meeting of the American Surgical Association
12. Bell RH Jr (2009) Why Johnny cannot operate. Surgery 146:533–542
13. Gawande AA (2001) Creating the educated surgeon in the 21st century. Am J Surg 181:551–556

Index

L. Bonavina (ed.), *Innovation in Esophageal Surgery*,
DOI 10.1007/978-88-470-2469-4, © Springer-Verlag Italia 2012

Q

R

S

T

V

GPSR Compliance

The European Union's (EU) General Product Safety Regulation (GPSR) is a set of rules that requires consumer products to be safe and our obligations to ensure this.

If you have any concerns about our products, you can contact us on ProductSafety@springernature.com

In case Publisher is established outside the EU, the EU authorized representative is:

Springer Nature Customer Service Center GmbH
Europaplatz 3
69115 Heidelberg, Germany

Batch number: 10683152

Printed by Printforce, the Netherlands